The Individualized Music Therapy Assessment Profile

of related interest

Multimodal Psychiatric Music Therapy for Adults, Adolescents, and Children
A Clinical Manual
Third Edition
Michael D. Cassity and Julia E. Cassity
ISBN 978 1 84310 831 3

A Comprehensive Guide to Music Therapy
Theory, Clinical Practice, Research and Training
Tony Wigram, Inge Nygaard Pedersen and Lars Ole Bonde
ISBN 978 1 84310 083 5

Receptive Methods in Music Therapy
Techniques and Clinical Applications for Music Therapy Clinicians, Educators and Students
Denise Grocke and Tony Wigram
Foreword by Cheryl Dileo
ISBN 978 1 84310 413 1

Improvisation
Methods and Techniques for Music Therapy Clinicians, Educators, and Students
Tony Wigram
Foreword by Professor Kenneth Bruscia
ISBN 978 1 84310 048 7

Filling a Need While Making Some Noise
A Music Therapist's Guide to Pediatrics
Kathy Irvine Lorenzato
Foreword by Kay Roskam
ISBN 978 1 84310 819 4

Interactive Music Therapy in Child and Family Psychiatry
Clinical Practice, Research and Teaching
Amelia Oldfield
Foreword by Dr Joanne Holmes
ISBN 978 1 84310 444 5

Roots of Musicality
Music Therapy and Personal Development
Daniel Perret
Foreword by Colwyn Trevarthen
ISBN 978 1 84310 336 2

Music Therapy with Children and their Families
Edited by Amelia Oldfield and Claire Flower
Foreword by Vince Hesketh
ISBN 978 1 84310 581 7

The Individualized Music Therapy Assessment Profile
IMTAP

Holly Tuesday Baxter, Julie Allis Berghofer, Lesa MacEwan, Judy Nelson, Kasi Peters, and Penny Roberts

Foreword by Ronald M. Borczon

Jessica Kingsley Publishers
London and Philadelphia

First published in 2007
by Jessica Kingsley Publishers
116 Pentonville Road
London N1 9JB, UK
and
400 Market Street, Suite 400
Philadelphia, PA 19106, USA

www.jkp.com

Copyright © Holly Tuesday Baxter, Julie Allis Berghofer, Lesa MacEwan, Judy Nelson,
Kasi Peters, and Penny Roberts 2007
Foreword copyright © Ronald M. Borczon 2007

All rights reserved. No part of this publication may be reproduced in any material form (including photocopying or storing it in any medium by electronic means and whether or not transiently or incidentally to some other use of this publication) without the written permission of the copyright owner except in accordance with the provisions of the Copyright, Designs and Patents Act 1988 or under the terms of a licence issued by the Copyright Licensing Agency Ltd, Saffron House, 6–10 Kirby Street, London EC1N 8TS. Applications for the copyright owner's written permission to reproduce any part of this publication should be addressed to the publisher.

Warning: The doing of an unauthorised act in relation to a copyright work may result in both a civil claim for damages and criminal prosecution.

All pages marked ✔ may be photocopied for personal use with this program, but may not be reproduced for any other purpose without the permission of the publisher.

Library of Congress Cataloging in Publication Data
A CIP catalog record for this book is available from the Library of Congress

British Library Cataloguing in Publication Data
A CIP catalogue record for this book is available from the British Library

ISBN 978 1 84310 866 5

Library of Congress Cataloging-in-Publication Data

The individualized music therapy assessment profile : IMTAP / Holly Tuesday Baxter ... [et al.] ; foreword by Ronald M. Borczon.
   p. cm.
Includes bibliographical references and index.
   ISBN-13: 978-1-84310-866-5 (pbk. : alk. paper) 1. Music therapy--Testing. I. Baxter, Holly Tuesday. II. Title: IMTAP.

ML3920.I47 2007
615.8'51540287--dc22

2007013568

Printed and bound in the United States by
Thomson-Shore, Inc.

Contents

Foreword by Ronald M. Borczon	9
Acknowledgments	11
Disclaimer	12

Chapter 1: Overview of the IMTAP — 13

- Purpose — 13
- Benefits and features — 13
- Administration time — 14
- User qualifications — 15

Chapter 2: Rationale for the Use of Music Therapy as an Assessment Protocol — 17

- Why music therapists assess — 17
- The need for a specific music therapy assessment — 18
- Unique qualities of the music therapy assessment — 19
- Summary — 20

Chapter 3: History and Development of the IMTAP — 21

- History — 21
- Item development — 21
- Domains and sub-domains — 22
  - Gross motor (GM) 22 – Fine motor (FM) 22 – Oral motor (OM) 22 – Sensory (SEN) 22 – Receptive communication/auditory perception (RC) 23 – Expressive communication (EC) 23 – Cognitive (COG) 23 – Emotional (EMO) 23 – Social (SOC) 23 – Musicality (MUS) 24
- Scoring system — 24

Chapter 4: Administration Instructions — 25

General considerations — 25

Age considerations and interpretation of scores — 25

Establishing a rapport — 26

Planning the assessment sessions — 26

The assessment process — 26

> Step one: the intake form 26 – Step two: the cover sheet 28 – Step three: the session outline 28 – Step four: data collection 28 – Step five: computing final scores 30 – Step six: reviewing cross-domain skills 31 – Step seven: the summary sheet 34 – Step eight: goals and objectives form 34 – Step nine: graphing 34

Chapter 5: The IMTAP Quantification Module — 37

Overview — 37

Preparation — 37

> Step one: skill selection 37 – Step two: the observe/record period 38 – Step three: selecting a time cueing system 38 – Step four: scoring symbols 38

Data collection — 39

> Step one: preparing the tally sheet 39 – Step two: recording and observing 39 – Step three: tallying scores 40

Chapter 6: Skill Definitions — 43

Gross motor skills (GM) — 43

> A. Fundamentals 43 – B. Perceptual/visual/psycho motor 44

Fine motor skills (FM) — 45

> A. Fundamentals 45 – B. Strumming 47 – C. Autoharp/Q Chord 47 – D. Guitar/dulcimer 48 – E. Piano 48 – F. Pitched percussive/mallet 50

Oral motor skills (OM) — 50

> A. Fundamentals 50 – B. Air production 51

Sensory skills (SEN) — 52

> A. Fundamentals 52 – B. Tactile 52 – C. Proprioceptive 53 – D. Vestibular 54 – E. Visual 55 – F. Auditory 56

Receptive communication/auditory perception (RC) — 57

> A. Fundamentals 57 – B. Direction following 57 – C. Musical changes 58 – D. Singing/vocalizing 59 – E. Rhythm 60

Expressive communication (EC)   61
    A. Fundamentals 61 – B. Non-vocal communication 61 – C. Vocalizations 62 –
    D. Spontaneous vocalizations 62 – E. Verbalizations 63 – F. Relational
    communication 63 – G. Vocal idiosyncrasies 64

Cognitive skills (COG)   65
    A. Fundamentals 65 – B. Decision making 66 – C. Direction following 66 –
    D. Short-term recall/sequencing 67 – E. Long-term recall 67 – F. Academics 68

Emotional skills (EMO)   71
    A. Fundamentals 71 – B. Differentiation/expression 71 – C. Regulation 71 –
    D. Self-awareness 72

Social skills (SOC)   73
    A. Fundamentals 73 – B. Participation 74 – C. Turn-taking 75 – D. Attention 76 –
    E. Direction following 77 – F. Relationship skills 77

Musicality (MUS)   79
    A. Fundamentals 79 – B. Tempo 80 – C. Rhythm 82 – D. Dynamics 84 – E. Vocal
    85 – F. Perfect and relative pitch 86 – G. Creativity and development of musical
    ideas 87 – H. Music reading 90 – I. Accompaniment 91

Chapter 7:   Case Studies   93

Case study 1: Neil   93
    Background 93 – Intake 93 – Assessment planning 94

Session 1   94
    Activities 94 – Musicality domain (MUS) 95 – Social domain (SOC) 97 – Session
    1 summary 98

Session 2   98
    Activities 98 – Musicality domain (MUS) 99 – Social domain (SOC) 100 –
    Session 2 summary 101

Session 3   101
    Activities 101 – Musicality domain (MUS) 102 – Social domain (SOC) 103 –
    Session 3 summary 104

IMTAP summary (Neil)   104

Case study 2: Timothy   108
    Background 108 – Intake 108 – Assessment planning 109 – Fine motor domain
    (FM) 111 – Receptive communication/auditory perception domain (RC) 112 –
    Expressive communication domain (EC) 114 – Cognitive domain (COG) 115 –
    Sensory domain (SEN) 116 – Social domain (SOC) 117 – Emotional domain
    (EMO) 119 – Musicality domain (MUS) 120

IMTAP summary (Timothy)   122

Chapter 8: The IMTAP Software and CD-ROM 127

Installing the IMTAP software 127
System requirements 127 – Installing on a Windows system 127 – Installing on a Macintosh system 128

Using the IMTAP software 128
Entering client records 129 – Viewing and printing client records 129 – Exporting Contact Information 130 – Conducting a client intake 130 – Recording assessment data 130 – Goals and objectives 132 – The Report Menu 133 – Printing 133

Technical support 134

Appendix A: IMTAP forms 135
Intake Form

Cover Sheet

Session Outline

Domain Forms

Gross Motor (GM) – Fine Motor (FM) – Oral Motor (OM) – Sensory (SEN) – Receptive Communication/Auditory Perception (RC) – Expressive Communication (EC) – Cognitive (COG) – Emotional (EMO) – Social (SOC) – Musicality (MUS)

Summary Form

Goals and Objectives

Graph Form

Quantification Form

Appendix B: Music Reading Samples 141
IMTAP Music Sample Hii

IMTAP Music Sample Hiii

IMTAP Music Sample Hv

IMTAP Music Sample Hvii

IMTAP Music Sample Hix

References 147
Index 149

Foreword

When I started the Music Therapy Wellness Clinic at California State University, Northridge, in 1996, I hired one music therapist, Judy Nelson, MT-BC, and we operated out of a classroom in the CSUN Music Building. As of this writing there are five music therapists who are part of the clinic structure, each possessing her own unique background and style of music therapy. The clinic has moved to a wonderful space with two clinic rooms that have VHS and DVD recording capabilities so that every session can be documented, a waiting area, an office for the therapists, and one-way mirrors for easy observation of a session.

As the clinic transformed and grew, so did the method of doing business. Part of any therapeutic practice is data collection, ranging from assessments to termination reports. Our approach to assessment evolved to such an extent that it ultimately provided this text, which is the culmination of several years of research, trial and error, meetings, video review, and plain old hard work. Thus, the Individualized Music Therapy Assessment Profile (IMTAP) was born out of a creative process and designed to provide a holistic picture of the client as well as to discover the areas that music therapy could best address.

To understand one of the many reasons that this assessment may have a broad appeal is to understand that at its genesis is a group of music therapists that have diverse viewpoints, methodologies, and experiences, yet are all deeply committed to music therapy and the assessment process. I think it is important to understand the background of the authors in order to see the various specialties that were involved in this process. Julie Berghofer, RMT, is a Nordoff Robbins trained music therapist and brings a humanistic and improvisational viewpoint to this work. Penny Roberts, MT-BC, has her Masters Degree in Music Therapy from Florida State University and offers a strong research-based behavioral paradigm. Judy Nelson, MT-BC, has a Masters Degree in Speech Pathology. Lesa MacEwan, MT-BC, has a Masters Degree in Special Education. Holly Baxter, MT-BC, comes from a holistic view of music therapy and brings technical expertise to the team. And Kasi Peters, MT-BC, is well versed in the Greenspan approach of "Floor Time." It is because of the ability of these professionals to respect each other's viewpoints and work collaboratively that this assessment is comprehensive, logical, and, most importantly, truly functional for clinical application. Once again, I found that believing in the power of music for the betterment of the client can unite varied philosophical approaches and creative minds.

I am especially excited about the potential of the IMTAP to address the entire continuum of music therapy work. For the educator, teaching students how to use the IMTAP will enable them to come into a variety of settings with an advanced tool for setting treatment goals and planning music therapy sessions. With the learning of this assessment at the pre-professional level, new music therapists will also have at their command a wonderful marketing tool as they move into the professional world. For the practicing clinician, this assessment will provide a comprehensive look at their client's functioning level and, through the computer analysis, will facilitate professional documentation. For those involved in research, there are possibilities just waiting to be discovered that the IMTAP can help facilitate. Ultimately, however, it is the clients assessed through this tool who will be the greatest beneficiaries of its development; it will be their lives that will be affected through innovative musical interventions planned due to information gleaned from its use.

I have seen numerous assessments in my many years as a music therapist and, through the history of music therapy, assessment tools have become more refined. I believe that the IMTAP is a significant contribution to an age old profession that is constantly growing, changing, and, in a changing age, striving to keep in step with technological developments. I am hopeful that as you learn the process of utilizing this tool, you will be able to see and understand your clients at many different levels; and that through the music you bring, you will be better able to help them move forward in their lives and in the world.

Ronald M. Borczon, M.M., MT-BC
Director of Music Therapy
California State University, Northridge

Acknowledgments

The IMTAP team wishes to acknowledge the many friends and colleagues who encouraged and supported the development of this work and particularly the music therapists who participated by review and beta testing.

Our special thanks go to Dr Diane Cullinane, Barbara Else, Sarah Hadley, Madeline Lieber, Victoria Lowrie, John McCarthy, Dr Clifford Madsen, Carrie Nakamura, Erin Salez, and Eric Waldon.

Thank you, Ron Borczon, for your enthusiasm and assistance in this process and for sharing our intentions with your students.

Our appreciation goes to all the clients and their families at the CSUN Music Therapy Wellness Clinic; you continue to be our inspiration.

Finally, deepest thanks to our families—Aaron, Aedan, Conal, Charly, Chuck, Finn, Lucas, Mike, Molly Ann, Rob, and Zac.

Disclaimer

The IMTAP is intended for use by board-certified or registered music therapists or students and/or interns working under the direct supervision of a board-certified or registered music therapist. The user takes all responsibility for the content and process of the music therapy session. The user takes all responsibility for abiding by any and all applicable laws of confidentiality and patient rights. The IMTAP does not diagnose nor does its use in any way guarantee efficacy of the music therapy process.

Chapter 1

Overview of the IMTAP

Purpose

The Individualized Music Therapy Assessment Profile (IMTAP) was created for use in pediatric and adolescent settings and is a multi-level process of assessment, beginning with intake and ending with a computer-based graphing and report system which provides a clear profile of each client over time. The IMTAP assesses each client using therapist-planned structured and/or improvisational music therapy interventions which are evaluated to assess domains of functioning. This process results in detailed, easy-to-understand information on client functioning and identification of effective music therapy strategies.

The IMTAP may be used on a variety of levels: as a treatment plan for music therapy work; as a tool to develop goals and objectives; as a means to address and assess targeted skill sets; as an indicator of overall functioning; as a baseline for treatment; as a research method; and as a communication tool for parents and healthcare professionals. The IMTAP provides information on a wide range of functioning abilities with a variety of clientele, including individuals with multiple severe physical disabilities, communication disorders, autism, severe emotional disturbances, social impairments, learning disabilities, and many other challenges.

Benefits and features

The IMTAP is an easy step-by-step process which can be tailored for use on a variety of levels. Each piece of the IMTAP can be used independently, or all of the features can be used together to create an in-depth profile of an individual. For example, music therapists working in an acute care setting may choose to assess only a single domain, while clients being seen on a long-term basis may be best served by participating in the entire process with all ten domains being scored to provide a full profile of client functioning.

The IMTAP does not utilize prescribed activities or require the use of a specific music therapy methodology. Music therapists and music therapy students can use their own repertoire of methods and activities to conduct the assessment sessions.

The IMTAP consists of several components:

- The **IMTAP intake** is completed with the referring individual or the parent/guardian and used to pinpoint assessment domains and plan assessment sessions.

- The **IMTAP cover sheet** summarizes the intake data and indicates the domains to be assessed.

- The **IMTAP session outline form** is used to plan assessment sessions, allowing the clinician to plan activities which directly assess the domains indicated during the intake process.

- The **IMTAP domain scoring forms** collect data on ten domains of functioning: gross motor; fine motor; oral motor; sensory; receptive communication/auditory perception; expressive communication; cognitive; social; emotional; and musicality. Within each domain there are various sub-domains which further clarify client functioning.

- The **IMTAP summary sheet** provides a means to summarize assessment data, resulting in subsets of client strengths and needs to facilitate a deeper understanding of client abilities. The summary sheet also provides a useful format for discussions with parents, educators, and others interested in the music therapy process.

- The **IMTAP goals and objectives form** provides a clear process for creating goals and objectives to address client needs.

- The **IMTAP quantification module** provides a quantified replicable score on a single skill which can be used for research and documentation purposes.

- The **IMTAP computer software** allows the therapist to centralize client information, score the assessment electronically, create reports and graphs, and track progress.

All of the above forms are provided as PDF files on the CD-ROM or may be copied from Appendix A.

Administration time

The IMTAP is a step-by-step process. Conducting the IMTAP intake is the first step and involves a structured conversation with the referring individual. To gather substantial information, the assessor can expect to spend between 30 and 45 minutes talking with the referring individual. In using the IMTAP to assess clients who are already participating in music therapy sessions, the therapist may choose to skip this step.

Step two involves planning the assessment sessions, which includes selecting the appropriate IMTAP domain scoring forms and developing activities. This may take 30 minutes to an hour, depending on the assessor's preferences for session planning. It is recommended that the IMTAP be conducted over the course of three sessions, with at least 30 minutes per session. It is strongly suggested that sessions be videotaped, but it is not required.

Step three requires completing the domain scoring forms. This may be done directly after the session by means of therapist recall or involve an in-depth analysis of session recordings. Dependent upon the number of domains scored and the means for review, the assessor can expect to spend between 15 and 90 minutes completing and scoring the IMTAP domain scoring forms. The IMTAP computer software provides automated means to complete these tasks and may greatly reduce the total time needed for scoring.

User qualifications

The IMTAP is designed to be used by board certified or registered music therapists or music therapy students and interns under the direct supervision of a board certified or registered music therapist. Professionals in related fields are qualified to review and use the information gathered from the IMTAP.

Chapter 2

Rationale for the Use of Music Therapy as an Assessment Protocol

Why music therapists assess

The American Music Therapy Association (AMTA) delineates assessment as one of the general Standards of Clinical Practice (2005). Similarly, the recent reauthorization of the Individuals with Disabilities Education Act Amendments of 2004 (IDEA) and the No Child Left Behind Act of 2001 (NCLB) emphasize assessment as a significant component of accountability for children with disabilities. To comply with these current mandates, there is a greater need for music therapists to develop viable assessment tools (Chase 2004; Flowers *et al.* 2005).

Assessment can be defined as "the process of gathering data about an area of learning through tests, observations, work samples, or other means" (Gunning 2000, p.487). It is necessary to assess the client's current level of functioning, needs, strengths, and preferences to develop an appropriate therapeutic program that targets the necessary skills for the client to learn to optimally function in the important environments of his/her life (Downing 1996; Orelove and Sobsey 1996; Westling and Fox 2004).

Accountability can be defined as the responsibility for how clients are making progress from their experiences (Elliott *et al.* 1998). Evaluation of client progress is essential for determining if the client is acquiring, maintaining, and generalizing targeted skills. Additionally, progress in these areas can be an indicator for effective therapeutic approaches and if any changes are required (Westling and Fox 2004).

The need for a specific music therapy assessment

As the music therapy profession has developed over the last two decades, music therapists have increasingly found themselves playing an integral role in interdisciplinary teams in a variety of professional settings (Davis, Gfeller, and Thaut 1999). While professions such as occupational therapy and speech therapy have produced formal published assessments, the field of music therapy has not (Chase 2004). This lack of formal published music therapy assessment tools has resulted in music therapists using assessments from other disciplines (Chase 2004; Gregory 2000). Many music therapists have adapted healthcare and/or educational assessments to utilize and observe music behavior (Chase 2004; Gregory 2000; Isenberg-Grzeda 1988). Wilson and Smith (2000) reported that more than half of music therapists working in school settings used self-created assessment tools; and the assessment tools that music therapists did use, whether self-created or published by discipline-specific fields other than music therapy, were not widely accessible to music therapists. However, using assessment instruments from other disciplines without the specific training to do so does not necessarily guarantee competency in administering these tests. Furthermore, using assessment tools not specifically designed for the music therapy profession may result in a lack of accurate assessment of the range of domains that music therapists serve or of specific music behaviors (Chase 2004; Gregory 2000; Scalenghe and Murphy 2000).

Without an assessment system in place, music therapy or any other field cannot achieve professional recognition (Cohen, Auerbach, and Katz 1978). Cohen *et al.* state: "the extent to which a therapist does or does not assess clients, and the type, degree, and quality of assessment performed, will influence attitudes and determine the role in which the therapist is viewed" (1978, p.92). Music therapists need to recognize the importance of assessment not only for the role it plays in driving music therapy intervention but also for the increase in professional credibility and integrity that will occur (Isenberg-Grzeda 1988; Lipe and York 1995). Given the existing practice of assessment in the field of music therapy, there appears to be a need for a systematic and formal music therapy assessment to validate sound practice and professional stature (Cohen *et al.* 1978; Gantt 2000). As federal mandates require greater accountability, music therapists must not rely on other professional assessments (Grant 1995). Rather, music therapists must develop and provide a music therapy assessment protocol, which parallels the standards of other professional assessment methodology to offer a unique perspective of client functioning to the interdisciplinary team (Grant 1995; Isenberg-Grzeda 1988).

> When music therapists develop an assessment tool that not only measures music-related functioning, but uses musical tasks and experiences as well as requiring a music therapist for its administration, our profession will have an independent identity among health care professionals. (Hintz 2000, p.36)

Not only is a formal music therapy assessment crucial for justification of music therapy intervention, it also lends credence to the field of music therapy as a viable therapeutic option (Scalenghe and Murphy 2000). While there is a lack of consensus within the music therapy profession regarding the need for a formalized assessment tool, there is an increased necessity due to the greater participation of music therapists in Individualized Education Programs (IEPs) and third-party funding (Grant 1995). For third-party funding sources to realize the need for music therapy services, music therapy assessment must be systematically implemented and consistent among all practitioners (Chase 2004).

Unique qualities of the music therapy assessment

One of the attributes of music is that it is motivating and fun (Alley 1979; Standley and Hughes 1997), whether it is the influence of auditory stimulation on the central nervous system (James *et al.* 1985) or that, in general, we simply associate music with positive experiences. Given the intrinsic properties of music and the plethora of techniques and tools available to music therapists (Thompson, Arnold, and Murray 1990), creating an assessment setting that is pleasurable may have potentially positive outcomes on client performance during the assessment process.

Another unique quality of a music therapy assessment is that music is a multi-sensory medium (Bruscia 1989). For example, while the auditory sense is being stimulated so can the tactile sense through the touch of a client's hand on drums; the visual sense when the client aims his/her mallet toward the drums; and the kinesthetic sense through the actual movement of reaching out to play the drums. As the client receives this multi-sensory stimulation, in turn, the client may provide the therapist with multi-sensory responses (Bruscia 1989). Furthermore, these multi-sensory responses may provide the music therapist with comprehensive assessment information spanning multiple domains.

An additional element to a music therapy assessment is the nonverbal aspect of music. The medium of music allows the therapist to transcend traditional verbal and/or visual symbolic systems (Wigram 2000). For example, during an improvisational musical experience, a preverbal or nonverbal client might engage in musical turn-taking with the therapist. This type of "dialogue" may be a nuance not immediately garnered through traditional verbal assessment procedures and may allow for the assessment of clients who are preverbal or nonverbal. Wigram (2000) states that through the flexibility of the improvisation process, not only can the areas of need within a client be observed, but the heretofore undiscovered strengths and abilities as well. Given the belief that musical ability is innate in each of us (Shuter-Dyson 1982), an assessment through the medium of music may utilize inherent abilities that clients with a range of disabilities may possess and that may not be easily recognizable through other assessment means.

The essential component in a music therapy assessment that does not exist in other discipline-specific assessment is, of course, the highly adaptable medium of music (Alley 1979). Through the universal experience of music, every individual can participate regardless of severity of disability (Gaston 1968; Nordoff and Robbins 1985). Given these realms of participation, multi-sensory input and response, the nonverbal aspect of music, and the motivating nature of this medium, music therapists have a great opportunity to perhaps see an additional and/or unique facet of client functioning and can certainly contribute a valid and beneficial perspective to the client's interdisciplinary team (Grant 1995; Isenberg-Grzeda 1988).

Summary

As federal mandates require greater accountability, music therapists must not rely only on other professional assessments (Grant 1995). Rather, music therapists must continue to develop and provide a music therapy assessment protocol, which parallels the standards of other professional assessment methodology in offering a unique perspective of client functioning to the interdisciplinary team (Grant 1995; Isenberg-Grzeda 1988). Not only can a comprehensive assessment tool promote music therapists' professional stature among other professions and justify a need for music therapy services, but such a tool also fosters consistency in language among practitioners as well as treatment and evaluation approaches. While all of these items are important, the most crucial rationale for a music therapy assessment tool is for the purpose of accurately determining who each client is, their unique strengths, areas of need and preferences in order to develop meaningful, appropriate treatment approaches that will support the client's functioning and enhance his/her quality of life to the best of our capabilities.

Chapter 3

History and Development of the IMTAP

History

The Individualized Music Therapy Assessment Profile was originally created to meet the needs of a music therapy clinic serving children and adolescents with a variety of diagnoses. Within the clinic, a team of six music therapists had identified the need for a reliable in-depth music therapy assessment protocol which met the requirements of third-party funding and would specifically address the need for quantitative data on non-musical domains within a musical environment. Additionally, the team required a common clinical language for use within and without the clinic. The IMTAP evolved over the course of five years from a simple narrative report to a detailed and systematic profile of 374 skills in ten separate domains.

Item development

To develop IMTAP test items, the authors completed a literature review of test instruments, standardized assessments and developmental surveys in the fields of music therapy, speech pathology, infant development, child development, occupational therapy, and school readiness. Reports and files of individuals seen in a clinical setting were also reviewed to expand the test criteria. Further items were developed in response to clients' needs, requests by other healthcare professionals and organizations, and to meet the requirements of the various music therapy modalities used by the clinicians. Test items were then reviewed by experts in the fields of music therapy, occupational therapy, speech pathology, psychology, and special education for further development and refinement.

Domains and sub-domains

Each IMTAP domain is divided into several sub-domains. These sub-domains help to clearly define which skill sets are being addressed within the broader domain. A music therapy client may score high in certain sub-domains and low in others. The IMTAP grading scale allows the therapist to document these differences. All domains begin with a "fundamentals" section and continue on to more highly developed sub-domains and skills. The ten IMTAP domains are outlined below.

Gross motor (GM)

Gross motor skills are those movements that take place in the large muscle groups or incorporate the whole body. The gross motor domain is sub-divided into two sub-domains: fundamentals and perceptual/visual/psycho motor. Fundamental skills assess right/left dominance, overall muscle tone, and how an individual moves his or her body within the music therapy experience. Perceptual/visual/psycho motor skills assess changes in movement and playing of instruments in response to musical stimuli.

Fine motor (FM)

Fine motor skills take place in the small muscle groups of the hands and fingers and are in coordination with the visual sense. Fundamental fine motor skills assess grasp, movement of fingers, and use of alternating hands. Assessment of the individual's abilities in strumming, autoharp/Q Chord, guitar/dulcimer, piano, and pitched percussive/mallet playing are also included in this domain.

Oral motor (OM)

The oral motor domain examines an individual's movement and coordination of the muscles and oral structures used in speech production and eating/drinking. These skills also serve to assess muscular strength, air production, and coordinated movements involved in vocalization and speech and are assessed in two sub-domains: fundamentals and air production.

Sensory (SEN)

The sensory domain assesses an individual's responses to, tolerance for, and integration of various sensory sub-domains through input received in the music therapy setting. The sub-domains assessed include tactile or sense of touch; proprioceptive or awareness of body in space; vestibular or balance; visual; and auditory.

Receptive communication/auditory perception (RC)

Receptive communication skills are examined to determine an individual's awareness, perception, discrimination, and response to various aspects of auditory stimuli and language in the environment. The sub-domains of musical changes, singing, and rhythm are used to examine responses to auditory input and communication. Responses to verbal direction within the music therapy setting are also assessed.

Expressive communication (EC)

The expressive communication domain assesses an individual's verbal and nonverbal communication skills within the music therapy setting including how gesture, vocalization, and verbalization are utilized by an individual, and to what degree. Relational communication and vocal idiosyncrasies are also examined in this domain.

Cognitive (COG)

Cognitive skills examine various aspects of the mental processes and functions of the individual that often contribute to success in educational environments. This domain includes the sub-domains of decision-making, direction-following, short-term recall/sequencing, long-term recall, and academics such as reading, counting and writing.

Emotional (EMO)

Emotional skills examine emotional or feeling states of the individual within the music therapy session. The various sub-domains which assess these skills are differentiation/expression, which assesses the individual's ability to express a range of emotional states; regulation, which assesses the individual's ability to respond within what is considered normal ranges of emotional expression and with appropriate control and modulation; and self-awareness of emotional states.

Social (SOC)

The social domain measures the ability of the individual to interact and communicate with others. These skills range from the basic fundamental skill of responding to one's name to the advanced relational skill of exploring external social relationships. Sub-domains include participation, turn-taking, attention, direction following, and relationship skills.

Musicality (MUS)

The musicality domain is intrinsic to the IMTAP and should be included in every assessment. This domain examines an individual's innate response to various musical mediums and his or her ability and desire to participate in each. Assessment of these areas acts as a prescriptive focus, allowing the music therapist to develop truly individualized interventions that involve the client in the musical experience directly. The fundamentals sub-domain assesses the individual's general interest in, reaction to, and enthusiasm for the music medium. Additional sub-domains include tempo; rhythm; dynamics; vocal; perfect and relative pitch; creativity and development of musical ideas; music reading; and accompaniment.

Scoring system

The IMTAP scoring system is based on two premises.

Premise one: Not all skills are of equal difficulty. As the IMTAP is working towards a profile of total client functioning, it identifies four levels of development. These are:

Level 1: Intrinsic skills, typically developed by 18 months of age and/or considered infant/toddler skills (i.e., explores instruments; anticipates own turn; attains full mouth closure).

Level 2: Basic skills, typically developed by 36 months of age and/or considered toddler skills (i.e., recalls name of instrument; established left/right hand dominance; plays in own tempo 1–4 measures).

Level 3: Learned skills, typically developed by 60 months of age and usually achieved by the conclusion of preschool (i.e., strums with whole hand and pulse; expresses emotions verbally; identifies letters A–G).

Level 4: Developed skills, typically developed after five years of age (i.e., reads lyrics; forms chords without prompting; plays multiples of basic beat).

Premise two: Within each level of skill development, each individual shall be assessed as to the consistency with which they demonstrate a skill. The IMTAP uses the initials NRIC, defined as:

N = never

R = rarely, under 50 percent

I = inconsistent, 50–79 percent

C = consistent, 80–100 percent.

The combination of these two premises allows for a wide variety of clientele to be assessed accurately and for a client profile to be created indicating the individual's areas of strength and difficulty and an overall level of general functioning.

Chapter 4

Administration Instructions

The IMTAP process consists of a variety of components which, together, create an in-depth profile of client functioning. Following an understanding of the various IMTAP components, the process may be tailored to meet the needs of the individual music therapist or music therapy setting. The administration instructions outline the use and purpose of each step in the IMTAP process.

All of the IMTAP forms may be found in Appendix A of this book as well as on the CD-ROM. The CD-ROM also includes a complete IMTAP software program which automates data collection, scoring, and graphing. The IMTAP is protected by all applicable copyright laws and the included forms and materials may be copied for use only by the single purchaser of this book.

General considerations

It is recommended that assessment sessions be administered in the same location throughout the assessment process in order to promote consistency and decrease anxiety on the part of the client. Planning of the assessment session using the IMTAP intake form and session outline form will allow the therapist to focus on the materials and activities which will be most conducive to thorough data collection. The authors suggest removing all materials except those necessary to conduct the session, to minimize distraction and promote on-task behaviors. In addition, it is suggested that sessions be recorded for ease and reliability in scoring. It is helpful to prepare any recording equipment such as video cameras or DVD recorders prior to the arrival of the client and start of the session.

Age considerations and interpretation of scores

The IMTAP can be tailored for use on a variety of levels and ages. With regard to age considerations, although various skills in the IMTAP have been correlated to published developmental assessments and other protocols, the IMTAP assessment is not standardized by age or age range. As a criterion-based assessment, the information resulting from the IMTAP process does not serve as a comparison of one client to another, but rather provides a deeper understanding of client functioning and the ability to track progress over time. As such, a young client would not be expected to achieve high scores on most domains or sub-domains. Rather than interpreting final score results independently, trends should be noticed as the client profile becomes apparent over several domains.

Establishing a rapport

It is important to begin establishing a rapport from the first contact with the client's representative, either when adding the client to a waiting list or during the intake. It may be helpful to begin by sharing information regarding the therapist's experience, training, approach, and general therapeutic setting before moving on to soliciting information. When asking for information, both client-age and diagnosis-appropriate language should be used. It may be helpful to begin with general questions regarding a specific domain and proceed with more detailed inquiries as the need becomes apparent. This initial contact should not be rushed, as this may be the parent/guardian's first exposure to music therapy, and certainly to the therapist and his/her organization. The parent/guardian may also need assurance on the procedure, location, and environment, as well as general education on music therapy.

Planning the assessment sessions

It is immensely helpful to visually record all sessions for review. It is suggested that three assessment sessions be utilized to fully complete the IMTAP. However, this is only a guideline, as fewer or more sessions may be necessary to cover all pertinent domains.

Clients who are seen for only one or two sessions may require a more focused assessment utilizing one or two IMTAP domains. The IMTAP may be used in this way to provide concise and immediate assessment in acute care situations.

The assessment process

Step one: the intake form

The IMTAP intake form is structured as a conversation with the referring individual, parent, or guardian and is a useful tool for planning the focus of music therapy assessment sessions. However, use of this form is not a requirement. In fact, when assessing a current client with whom a therapist has already been working, the IMTAP intake form would probably not be utilized. In such a case, the therapist may proceed directly to planning the assessment session.

The IMTAP intake form begins with a general information section detailing the child's history as well as musical aptitude and exposure.

The next section of the intake form is organized by domain. Completion of the domain sections assists in identifying which domains of functioning require attention in the assessment sessions. During the intake conversation, parents/guardians may be unsure of or withhold information regarding client behavior, level of functioning, or history. If an area of conversation is perceived to be difficult or lacking in sufficient information, it is advisable to check the left box of the applicable section, indicating that this domain is to be assessed.

1. Complete the client information section of the form including the name of the referring individual as well as that of the interviewee, who may be different from the referrer.

2. After entering the intake date and client's birth date, subtract the year, month, and day of the birth date from the year, month, and day of the intake date to arrive at the client's chronological age.

3. Proceed through the general information section of the intake during your conversation with the referring individual marking "yes" or "no" as appropriate.

4. Proceed through the individual domain sections during your conversation with the referring individual marking "yes" or "no" as appropriate.

5. Space is provided for notes on each question as well as for items or areas which may not have been covered during the intake process. A space is also provided for the therapist's perceptions or initial areas of interest.

6. After completing the intake interview, refer to the completed intake form noticing any indications in the left hand "yes/no" shaded column of the domain sections. Any indications in this shaded column cue the therapist to assess this domain.

7. On the final sheet of the intake form, complete the intake summary checkboxes, checking the domains in which indications were made in the left hand/shaded column of the domain sections above.

You will notice that the musicality box is checked for you. It is suggested that musicality always be assessed, not due to any requirement or desire for a client to possess musical aptitude but rather as a means to identify effective music therapy strategies.

Step two: the cover sheet

1. Complete the client information section of the IMTAP cover sheet form.

2. After entering the assessment date and client's birth date, subtract the year, month, and day of the birth date from the year, month, and day of the assessment date to arrive at the client's chronological age.

3. Indicate which domains will be assessed in the appropriate checkboxes.

4. Copy or print the corresponding IMTAP domain scoring sheets from Appendix A or the accompanying software.

Step three: the session outline

The optional IMTAP session outline form may be used to plan musical interventions for each domain you will be assessing. This is organized not by activity, but rather by the domain to be assessed. This form may be used to list activities, songs, instruments, materials, and other necessary considerations needed for your assessment sessions.

1. Complete the client and assessment information section of the IMTAP session outline form.

2. Indicate which domains will be assessed in the appropriate checkboxes.

3. List activities, songs, instruments, materials, or other considerations for each domain that is to be assessed. A single activity may be listed in numerous domains.

Step four: data collection

Scoring

Sessions are scored according to the consistency with which the client demonstrates the skills in each domain and sub-domain. The levels of consistency are as follows:

N = never

R = rarely, under 50 percent

I = inconsistent, 50–79 percent

C = consistent, 80–100 percent

The NRIC system may be used one of two ways: estimated or tallied. Estimated scores are typically used when the results are purely for the therapist's use in planning and tracking treatment. Tallying scores involves counting the number of opportunities presented and dividing into the number of times the skill was demonstrated, indicating the level of consistency according to this percentage. For example, in scoring the skill "Looks for hidden or dropped object" (COG, Aii), if an object was hidden four times and the client searched for it twice the resulting percentage would be 50, indicating an "Inconsistent (50–79%)" response to this skill. Use of either estimated or tallied scoring should be determined by the therapist's resources and clinical needs.

The IMTAP may be partially completed and referred to between assessment sessions in order to assist in planning future sessions.

Non-assessed sub-domains and skills

Each sub-domain has the option of being marked "N/A" if it was not assessed by the therapist. This should be used only for sub-domains for which there was not time or sufficient resources to assess. For example, Fine Motor E (Piano) may be marked as "N/A" if a piano was not available. "N/A" should not be used if the sub-domain was not assessed due to client functioning level. "N/A" may not be used for single skills within a sub-domain.

If a particular skill is clearly above the individual's level of functioning it should be scored N for "Never." For example, in the fine motor domain, an individual who receives an N on "Uses palmar grasp" (FM, Aii) would also receive an N on "Sustains palmar grasp with dominant hand," (FM, Aix) a later skill which measures a higher level of development.

Conversely, if a skill is clearly below the individual's level of functioning it should be scored C for "Consistent." For example, in the strumming sub-domain of fine motor, if an individual scores C on "Strums with pick and pulse" (FM, Bvi), the therapist would not then ask the individual to demonstrate strumming with a whole hand, an earlier development of the same skill. The therapist would instead mark "Whole hand" (FM, Bi) with a C.

For some individuals, an entire sub-domain may be above or below their level of functioning. For example, the music reading sub-domain of musicality may be clearly above an individual's level of functioning, or the fundamentals sections of many domains may be clearly below an individual's level of functioning. In such cases, each item should be scored C or N.

Each domain includes a fundamentals sub-domain. This sub-domain must be assessed and cannot be marked "N/A." Consistent assessment of these skills allows for continuity in scoring over time and throughout the assessment process.

Step five: computing final scores

First compute the sub-domain raw score:

1. Calculate the raw score for each column of the assessed sub-domains by adding the numbers indicated next to the C, I, R, or N for each skill and entering the total at the bottom of the column (Figure 4.1; bold indications show scoring).

2. Total the raw scores for each column to arrive at the sub-domain raw score.

F. Pitched Percussive/Mallet							n/a ☐
i.	Plays small instrument with mallet when presented	N_0	R_1	I_2	**C_3**		
ii.	Plays any note with mallet	N_0	R_1	I_2	**C_3**		
iii.	Plays isolated note with mallet from multiple choices		N_0	R_2	I_3	**C_4**	
iv.	Plays mallet with strike and retract motion		N_0	R_2	**I_3**	C_4	
v.	Sequences simple pattern of notes			**N_0**	R_3	I_4	C_5
	Column Totals:	0	0	9	4	0	
	Add Column Totals to calculate **Raw Score**:					13	

Figure 4.1

Next compute the sub-domain and domain final scores:

1. Transfer raw scores from each sub-domain to the Summary box located after the final sub-domain.

2. In the Summary box, place a check in the "N/A" column for any sub-domains which were not assessed.

3. Transfer the client's score for each assessed sub-domain to the Raw Score column and divide by the total possible to compute the sub-domain final score.

4. To compute the domain raw score, add the numbers in the Raw Score column.

5. Add the numbers provided in the Possible column for all sub-domains which were assessed. Enter the total in the final row of the Possible column. Do not include sub-domains which were not assessed.

6. Divide the domain raw score by the total domain possible to compute the domain final score (Figure 4.2).

Summary

Sub-Domain	n/a	Raw Score		Possible		Final Score
A. Fundamentals		35	÷	39	=	90 %
B. Strumming		20	÷	27	=	74 %
C. Autoharp/Omnichord	✓		÷	15	=	%
D. Guitar/Dulcimer	✓		÷	42	=	%
E. Piano		17	÷	41	=	41 %
F. Pitched Percussive/Mallet		13	÷	19	=	68 %
Domain Total (Fine Motor)		85	÷	126	=	67 %

Figure 4.2

Step six: reviewing cross-domain skills

A number of IMTAP skills are defined as cross-domain skills, or skills which appear in more than one domain. A low score on a cross-domain skill may indicate a need to assess the corresponding domain(s). These skills are indicated on the IMTAP domains with a "*CD*" notation. An alphabetical list of these skills and their corresponding domains and sub-domains follows.

Adapts playing to match meter changes

> Gross motor – perceptual/visual/psycho motor
> Musicality – tempo

Adapts playing to match tempo changes

> Gross motor – perceptual/visual/psycho motor
> Musicality – tempo

Answers closed (yes/no) questions

> Cognitive – decision making
> Expressive communication – relational communication

Conscious body movement in tempo

> Gross motor – perceptual/visual/psycho motor
> Musicality – tempo

Demonstrates awareness of gross dynamic changes

> Musicality – dynamics
> Receptive communication/auditory perception – musical changes

Demonstrates awareness of gross tempo changes

    Musicality – tempo
    Receptive communication/auditory perception – musical changes

Demonstrates awareness of sound vs. silence

    Receptive communication/auditory perception – fundamentals
    Sensory – auditory

Demonstrates understanding of rules and structures

    Cognitive – fundamentals
    Social – fundamentals

Follows one-step verbal direction

    Cognitive – direction following
    Receptive communication/auditory perception – direction following
    Social – direction following

Follows simple musical cues

    Cognitive – direction following
    Receptive communication/auditory perception – direction following
    Social – direction following

Follows two-step verbal direction

    Cognitive – direction following
    Receptive communication/auditory perception – direction following
    Social – direction following

Imitates intermediate rhythmic pattern

    Musicality – rhythm
    Receptive communication/auditory perception – rhythm

Imitates simple rhythmic pattern

    Musicality – rhythm
    Receptive communication/auditory perception – rhythm

Plays in tempo of therapist 1–4 measures

    Gross motor – perceptual/visual/psycho motor
    Musicality – tempo
    Receptive communication/auditory perception – rhythm

Plays simple accompaniment using chord chart

    Cognitive – academics
    Fine motor – autoharp/Q Chord
    Musicality – music reading

Reads treble clef notation

    Cognitive – academics
    Musicality – music reading

Sings pitched melody accurately

    Musicality – vocal
    Receptive communication/auditory perception – singing/vocalizing

Sustains activity-length attention span

    Cognitive – fundamentals
    Social – attention

Tolerates putting mouthpiece to lips

    Oral motor – air production
    Sensory – tactile

Transcribes musical ideas using symbols or notation

    Cognitive – academics
    Musicality – creativity and development of musical ideas

Unconscious body movements in tempo

    Gross motor – perceptual/visual/psycho motor
    Musicality – tempo

Unconscious vocalizations in tonality

    Musicality – vocal
    Receptive communication/auditory perception – singing/vocalizing

Vocalizes in response to particular musical style/idiom

    Musicality – vocal
    Receptive communication/auditory perception – singing/vocalizing

Step seven: the summary sheet

The IMTAP summary sheet provides a general format for reviewing the music therapy assessment with the individual's parents or guardians. After completing scoring of the IMTAP, the therapist should review the results to discern which domains or sub-domains qualify as strengths or needs. Typically, the top-scoring sub-domains or areas which did not require assessment would be identified as strengths. Lower-scoring sub-domains or areas which are either inhibiting or minimizing the potential of the individual's ability to participate in daily activities may be identified as needs. As the IMTAP summary is intended as an informal means to communicate a condensed client profile, not all assessed sub-domains would be listed on this form. Strengths and needs may be outlined in either bullet point or narrative fashion.

Step eight: goals and objectives form

Use the goals and objectives form to relate your client's goals directly to the IMTAP categories you have identified and assessed. The page number and number of pages have been left blank at the bottom right of the form for your use in copying as needed.

Step nine: graphing

Creating a domain profile graph

The IMTAP graph is the final step in providing a complete profile of client functioning and provides a clear, visual representation of the various domains and sub-domains assessed. The graph is shaded for ease of viewing and assistance in visualizing trends in scoring. Scores in the darkest shaded portion are in the highest level of functioning and scores in the non-shaded area are in the lowest level of functioning. This, however, is not an absolute indicator of client needs or strengths. Determinations of client need should be based on peaks and valleys shown by the graphing process. For example, a very young child may not score above 60 percent in any domains. However, if four of the child's domain scores are in the 50–60 percent range while a fifth domain scores 95 percent, this domain would clearly show a strength in that area. Additionally, if a sixth domain scored at 5 percent, this would demonstrate a strong need in this area (Figure 4.3).

1. Enter the client name, date of birth, and assessment date on the IMTAP graph form.

2. Enter a title for the graph. This may be "Overall Functioning" or "All Domains."

3. Check the Domain Profile box.

4. In the column labeled Domain/Sub-Domain, list the domains which were assessed.

5. To the right of each domain, place a mark in the approximate position corresponding to the score for the domain as determined in the Domain Summary box at the conclusion of each domain's scoring sheets. Use the score markings along the bottom edge of the graph for reference.

6. Connect the markings using a straight edge (see Figure 4.3).

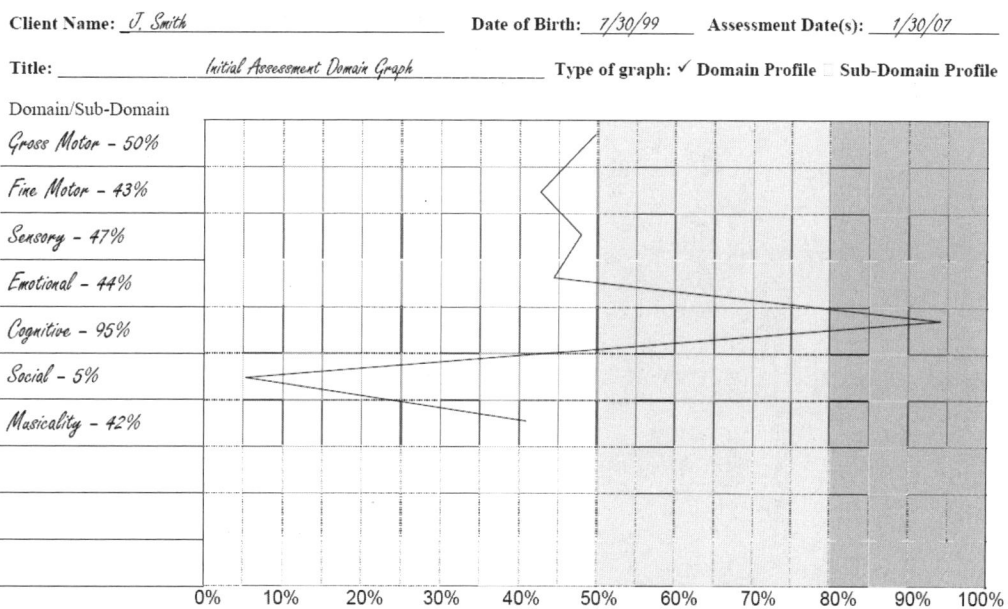

Figure 4.3

Creating a sub-domain profile graph

For domains of interest, you may wish to also plot the sub-domain scores. This can be particularly useful in domains with a large number of sub-domains, such as musicality or expressive communication. In these larger domains, the domain score alone does not provide a complete picture of client functioning and further detail may be useful. For example, a client who receives a score of 51 percent in the musicality domain can have a range of 85 percent to 15 percent in the various sub-domains of musicality. Plotting these sub-domains is very useful to pinpointing exactly which areas require further support and development.

1. Enter the client name, date of birth, and assessment date on the IMTAP graph form.

2. Enter a title for the graph. This should be the name of the domain.

3. Check the Sub-Domain Profile box.

4. In the column labeled Domain/Sub-Domain, list the sub-domains which were assessed.

5. To the right of each sub-domain, place a mark in the approximate position corresponding to the score for the sub-domain as determined in the Domain Summary box at the conclusion of each domain's scoring sheets. Use the score markings along the bottom edge of the graph for reference.

6. Connect the markings using a straight edge.

The IMTAP graph may be used creatively to compare and provide assessment data. Various colors or symbols can be used in order to plot progress over time or to compare assessment data.

Chapter 5

The IMTAP Quantification Module

Overview

The quantification module is provided for data collection in research, third-party funding, and documentation. It is useful in documenting progress to parents/guardians, educators, healthcare professionals, and others who may need visual and/or numerical representations of the music therapy intervention. In these and other situations, it is essential to quantify therapeutic results by replicable means.

The IMTAP quantification module complements the standard NRIC scoring system by utilizing the observance of a single skill to provide statistical data. Observation of the single skill provides a sample of behavior, which is then converted into a percentage. During the quantification process, the clinician alternates between observing the client and recording data. This is a documented method of data collection which results in a replicable numerical score.

Recorded or live sessions may be observed for data collection. However, if a live session is utilized, it is suggested that an additional reliability observer be present to simultaneously collect data.

Preparation

Step one: skill selection

Quantification may be most useful in documenting specific skills or skill sets, such as the fundamentals sub-domain of each IMTAP domain. It is judicious to choose skills that leave little or no room for debate or interpretation. That is, it is more appropriate to measure "Reaches to touch/play instrument" (GM, Aiii) than to attempt to measure his/her endeavor to transcribe musical ideas using symbols or notation (MUS, Gxiii).

In addition, it is essential to identify the exact behavior you wish to measure before you begin quantification.

Step two: the observe/record period

Precise data recording is the key to providing accurate statistical results. With this in mind, the challenge of observing and recording data can be daunting. This method of data collection utilizes a dedicated period for observation only, followed by a dedicated recording period.

In the following example we will use a five-second observe, five-second record structure. Deciding on the time period is an important step in preparing for data collection. If the behavior you are observing occurs often or at a rapid pace during the activity (e.g., a very excited client or frequent occurrence of the skill), you may wish to use a short time period, such as a three-second observe and record. If the behavior is slow, such as a client with very slow movements responding at a slow tempo and with significant delay, you may wish to extend the time allotted for observe and record. *However, the period of observation and record is not to be adjusted after tallying has begun.*

Step three: selecting a time cueing system

An electronic device is imperative to assist with quantification. If you have access to a tape recorder or other recording device, it is suggested to record a loop of "Observe" and "Record" at the time allotment you have chosen. If this is prohibitive, a metronome with differentiated downbeat may be used. A visual timing device can be used, but this is not suggested as it can distract from the observation period in which all attention should be focused on the client. This is a personal choice and either will yield the same results.

In this example, a five-second observe/record period was chosen. A recorded loop was made with the verbal cue of "Observe" to begin the tape. At five-second intervals, the cues "Record" and then, five seconds later, "Observe" were repeated for a time sufficient to collect data.

Step four: scoring symbols

Before beginning, become familiar with the symbols and what they represent:

+ = desired skill demonstrated

V = desired skill not demonstrated due to verbal distraction (e.g., client sings/speaks to therapist or others when cued to perform a nonverbal skill)

M = desired skill not demonstrated due to motor distraction or different action (e.g., client is flapping when cued to strike the drum or client jumps when instructed to sit)

O = desired behavior not demonstrated due to no interaction

A = N/A, when it was not possible for client to demonstrate skill or unable to be measured (e.g., dropping the instrument or client moves out of view).

Data collection

Step one: preparing the tally sheet

On the IMTAP quantification tally sheet, complete the client name, date, and reliability observer name (if any).

The first column of the form contains time measurements for you to accurately track your quantification. Fill in this box with the time stamp from the recording you are watching. In this example (Figure 5.1), the music therapist began observing the activity when the time on the recording read 12:55.

| 1

12:55 | Obs | +V M

O A | Obs | +V M

O A | Obs | +V M

O A |

Figure 5.1

Fill in all subsequent first columns as you are able. Should there be an interruption in the data collection process, this will prevent starting again from the beginning.

Step two: recording and observing

As the clinician watches the session (with the device chosen to represent the observe and record periods), each symbol is marked only once, regardless of the number of times the behavior was demonstrated. For example, although the client demonstrated "Reaches to touch/play instrument" three times in one observe period, the + is marked a single time.

If the client did not demonstrate this behavior because he/she was distracted verbally (e.g., talking to oneself, talking to therapist, singing, etc.), slash through the V symbol to indicate a verbal distraction. If the client did not reach for the instrument because he/she was distracted with motor movements (flapping, hitting, etc.) the M symbol should be marked. Off-task behavior such as daydreaming, light gazing, refusal to cooperate, etc., would be marked using the O symbol. Lastly, the "N/A" may be used when the opportunity was not presented or could not be recorded (e.g., the client drops the mallet, the therapist stops the music to redirect, or the client moves out of view of the recorder).

While several behaviors may be recorded in any timeframe, slash only once per symbol. For example, if the client reaches to touch/play an instrument twice upon cue, but when cued again in the same observe timeframe asks the therapist for a new activity, this would be recorded as two slashes in the same box: one + for the demonstrated skill and one V to indicate a verbal distraction.

Record through the duration of the recording interval, recording no other behavior other than what was observed in the previous observation interval. As this system records a statistical sample of a behavior, only behaviors observed during the observation period are recorded. For example, if a client does not demonstrate the skill during the observation period, but then demonstrates the skill during the record period, no data is collected. *During the observe portion, look only at the recording; during the record portion, look only at the paper!*

Step three: tallying scores

1. Count the number of responses of each type and enter in the corresponding blank at the bottom of the tally sheet.

2. Enter the total number of boxes in the second blank.

3. Divide the first number by the second to arrive at your percentage.

4. Enter the result in the final blank space.

For example, if six boxes were completed and the client demonstrated the desired skill (+) in three of the boxes, the client demonstrated the desired skill 50 percent of the time (Figure 5.2).

The final percentage score indicates the percentage of time in which the client demonstrated the behavior or distraction. In Figure 5.3, the client demonstrated the desired skill 50 percent of the time and also demonstrated a verbal distraction 33 percent of the time. This is to be expected, as clients typically demonstrate various behaviors in the same observation period. The demonstration of one behavior does not preclude the presence of another.

This system results in a statistical representation of a sample of behavior. Each type of behavior can be considered as an independent indication of client functioning. Clients who demonstrate the desired skill 100 percent of the time may also have a need in the areas of verbal distraction, motor distraction, or off-task behavior. Significant changes in behavior may be observed as these percentages increase or decrease.

1 --:--	Obs	✓ V M O A	Obs	+ V M O A	Obs	+ V M O A
2 --:--	Obs	+ V M O A	Obs	✓ V M O A	Obs	✓ V M O A

+:   **3** / **6** = **50** %

Figure 5.2

1 --:--	Obs	✓ V M O A	Obs	+ ✓ M O A	Obs	+ V M O A
2 --:--	Obs	+ V M O A	Obs	✓ ✓ M O A	Obs	✓ V M O A

+:   **3** / **6** = **50** %

V: **2** / **6** = **33** %

M: _____ / _____ = _____ %

O: _____ / _____ = _____ %

A: _____ / _____ = _____ %

Figure 5.3

Chapter 6

Skill Definitions

Gross motor skills (GM)

A. Fundamentals

i. Moves spontaneously

Client independently moves without visual, verbal, musical, or physical prompting by therapist.

ii. Displays appropriate muscle tone during movement

Client demonstrates control and stability in posture and movement of large muscles when sitting, standing, walking, and/or dancing.

iii. Reaches to touch/play instrument

Client spontaneously reaches toward or touches instrument without physical assistance.

iv. Displays heel–toe gait

Client distributes weight from heel, through entire foot, to toe when walking. Does not exhibit walking on tip-toes or heels.

v. Displays even walking gait

Client walks with equal weight transfer, rhythm, and stride.

vi. Established left/right dominance

Client demonstrates use of one hand more than the other.

vii. Crosses body midline
Client moves arms and/or legs across vertical center of body to opposite side during task.

viii. Coordinates playing of two different instruments
Client plays two different instruments simultaneously or sequentially. Examples of instruments requiring gross motor movement include drums or cymbals.

B. Perceptual/visual/psycho motor

General definition. Perceptual/visual/psycho motor tasks are those that require information from the senses (aural, visual, tactile) to be perceived and acted upon and the motor activity directly related to or a result of mental processes. Examples include imitation of body movements or playing in tempo.

i. Demonstrates motor agitation
Client demonstrates motion without apparent purpose or function. Examples include tremor, pacing, wringing hands, tugging on clothes, etc.

ii. Unconscious body movements in tempo
Client demonstrates unintended or involuntary movement in tempo of music.

iii. Conscious body movements in tempo
Client demonstrates intended or voluntary movement in tempo of music.

iv. Moves in organized manner
Client demonstrates ability to plan, execute, and complete gross motor movements.

v. Movements are related to musical stimuli
Client responds to musical stimuli with observable body movement such as dancing, drumming, or swaying.

vi. Plays in tempo of therapist 1–4 measures
Client plays instrument matching the same tempo as the therapist for 1–4 measures.

SKILL DEFINITIONS – FINE MOTOR SKILLS

vii. Imitates gross motor movements of therapist
Client imitates gross motor movements in a musical or non-musical activity.

viii. Demonstrates ability to stop/go on cue
Client demonstrates ability to stop/go upon receiving a verbal, visual, auditory, musical, or physical prompt.

ix. Adapts playing in response to non-musical cues
Client demonstrates ability to change dynamics, tempo or instrument choices from non-musical cues.

x. Adapts playing to match dynamic changes
Client demonstrates ability to change dynamics from musical cue alone.

xi. Adapts playing to match tempo changes
Client demonstrates ability to change tempo from musical cue alone.

xii. Demonstrates ability to sequence two movements
Client produces two distinct cued movements in succession.

xiii. Demonstrates ability to sequence three or more movements
Client produces three distinct cued movements in succession.

xiv. Adapts playing to match meter changes
Client demonstrates ability to change meter from musical cue alone.

xv. Demonstrates ability to develop movement sequences
Client is able to independently expand upon a gross motor movement sequence.

Fine motor skills (FM)

A. Fundamentals

i. Displays use of both hands
Client uses both hands during music therapy activities.

ii. Uses palmar grasp
Client uses whole hand when grasping objects.

iii. Uses pincer grasp
Client uses the tips of the thumb and index finger to grasp objects.

iv. Holds object/instrument independently with one hand
Client holds object or instrument in one hand without assistance.

v. Holds object/instrument independently with two hands
Client holds single object or instrument in each hand without assistance.

vi. Established left/right hand dominance
Client demonstrates use of one hand more than the other.

vii. Forms shapes with fingers and/or isolates fingers during finger play activities
Client uses fingers to form shapes and/or uses individual fingers during finger play activities such as "Eeensy Weensy Spider," counting games, or "Twinkle, Twinkle."

viii. Plays instrument with alternating hands
Client uses both hands successively with or without an observable pattern.

ix. Sustains palmar grasp with dominant hand
Client is able to hold object in whole of dominant hand for a minimum of four consecutive seconds. If client does not have demonstrated left/right dominance, score this skill using right hand.

x. Sustains palmar grasp with non-dominant hand
Client is able to hold object in whole of non-dominant hand for a minimum of four consecutive seconds. If client does not have demonstrated left/right dominance, score this skill using left hand.

xi. Organizes alternating hands in playing
Client uses both hands successively with an observable motor pattern.

B. Strumming

i. Whole hand
Client uses index, middle, ring, and pinky finger together to strum instrument.

ii. Single finger
Client isolates one finger to strum instrument.

iii. Whole hand with pulse
Client uses index, middle, ring, and pinky finger together to strum instrument with a consistent emphasis on the beats of the music.

iv. Single finger with pulse
Client isolates one finger to strum instrument with a consistent emphasis on the beats of the music.

v. Strums with pick
Client holds pick between index finger and thumb to strum instrument.

vi. Strums with pick and pulse
Client holds pick between index finger and thumb to strum instrument with a consistent emphasis on the beats of the music.

C. Autoharp/Q Chord

i. Explores chord buttons
Client touches and pushes buttons without assistance.

ii. Depresses single button on cue
Client pushes button in response to visual, verbal, physical, or musical cue.

iii. Coordinates press and strum
Client pushes button with one hand while simultaneously strumming with the other hand.

iv. Plays simple accompaniment using chord chart

Client simultaneously pushes buttons and strums from chord chart of two or more chords.

D. Guitar/dulcimer

i. Forms chords with prompting

Client isolates fingers to place at least two fingers on specific frets/strings to create a recognizable chord. Prompts may include visual, verbal, or physical cues.

ii. Approximates simple chord positions

Client independently shapes fingers in the approximate form of a simple chord of at least two fingers such as E7, A major, and D major guitar chords or basic dulcimer chords.

iii. Forms chords in simple musical pattern

Client changes between two or more recognizable chords in a musical pattern.

iv. Forms chords in advanced musical pattern

Client changes between four or more recognizable chords in a musical pattern.

v. Plays using chord chart

Client independently forms and plays chords in correct sequence from chord chart.

vi. Plays individual strings

Client plays one string independent of other strings on instrument.

vii. Plays individual strings with pulse

Client plays one string independent of other strings on instrument with a consistent emphasis on the beats of the music.

E. Piano

i. Coordinates both hands

Client uses both hands simultaneously to play isolated keys.

ii. Uses fingers of dominant hand without splaying

Client manipulates fingers of dominant hand without rigidity or over-extension of finger span. If client does not have demonstrated left/right dominance, score this skill using right hand.

iii. Uses fingers of non-dominant hand without splaying

Client manipulates fingers of non-dominant hand without rigidity or over-extension of finger span. If client does not have demonstrated left/right dominance, score this skill using left hand.

iv. Uses single finger of dominant hand

Client isolates one finger of dominant hand to play keys. If client does not have demonstrated left/right dominance, score this skill using right hand.

v. Uses single finger of non-dominant hand

Client isolates one finger of non-dominant hand to play keys. If client does not have demonstrated left/right dominance, score this skill using left hand.

vi. Sequences multiple fingers on dominant hand

Client isolates at least two individual fingers on dominant hand to play keys in succession. If client does not have demonstrated left/right dominance, score this skill using right hand.

vii. Sequences multiple fingers on non-dominant hand

Client isolates at least two individual fingers on non-dominant hand to play keys in succession. If client does not have demonstrated left/right dominance, score this skill using left hand.

viii. Forms triads with dominant hand

Client isolates three fingers or two fingers and thumb of dominant hand to simultaneously play three different keys. If client does not have demonstrated left/right dominance, score this skill using right hand.

ix. Forms triads with non-dominant hand
Client isolates three fingers or two fingers and thumb of non-dominant hand to simultaneously play three different keys. If client does not have demonstrated left/right dominance, score this skill using left hand.

F. Pitched percussive/mallet
i. Plays small instrument with mallet when presented
Client grasps and uses mallet to play any small instrument which requires precision, such as tone bar, temple block, or glockenspiel.

ii. Plays isolated note with mallet from multiple choices
Client grasps and uses mallet to play a single note on pitched percussive instrument with multiple choices, such as xylophone or log drum.

iii. Plays mallet with strike and retract motion
Client grasps and uses mallet to play single note with strike and retract motion producing ringing tone from pitched percussive instrument.

iv. Sequences simple pattern of notes
Client grasps and uses mallet to play two or more notes in succession on a pitched percussive instrument.

Oral motor skills (OM)
A. Fundamentals
i. Demonstrates full range of motion when opening
Client is able to fully open mouth vertically beyond three fingers' width.

ii. Demonstrates full range of motion when smiling
Client is able to fully retract corners of mouth into recognizable smile.

iii. Demonstrates full range of motion when puckering
Client is able to compress lips and move them forward into a kissing posture.

iv. Attains full mouth closure
Client is able to close lips without a gap between upper and lower lip.

B. Air production

i. Tolerates putting mouthpiece to lips

Client places mouthpiece of instrument to lips without resistance or distress. Ability to tolerate may differ according to material of mouthpiece (i.e., wood, plastic, metal).

ii. Produces tone

Client produces audible sound via blowing through mouthpiece of instrument. Does not include humming through mouthpiece.

iii. Able to produce tone on cue

Client produces audible sound via blowing through mouthpiece of instrument when cued by therapist. Does not include humming through mouthpiece.

iv. Produces tone of one second or less

Client produces audible sound via blowing through mouthpiece of instrument of one second or less. Does not include humming through mouthpiece.

v. Produces tone of greater than one second

Client produces audible sound via blowing through mouthpiece of instrument of more than one second. Does not include humming through mouthpiece.

vi. Produces simple rhythmic pattern

Simple rhythmic patterns are defined as patterns of no more than one measure in length, in either duple or triple meter, using quarter and eighth values only. Can also include simple rhythmic patterns based on names starting on upbeat or first beat of bar. Does not include humming through mouthpiece.

vii. Integrates tone production and gross motor movement

Client produces tone while participating in gross motor movement such as walking.

viii. Integrates tone production and fine motor movement

Client produces tone while participating in fine motor movement. Examples include playing the recorder, slide whistle, or melodica.

Sensory skills (SEN)
A. Fundamentals

i. Integrates sensory input of two types
Client participates in activity which involves two types of sensory input, such as auditory and visual, or tactile and proprioceptive.

ii. Integrates multiple sensory input types
Client participates in activity which involves three types of sensory input, such as auditory, visual, and tactile.

B. Tactile

General definition. Tactile input is any information received from touch senses.

i. Seeks firm pressure
Seeking may take the form of participating in action or requesting action. Examples of firm pressure include rolling a cabasa on the body, placing therapist's hands on the body, or pressing the body against a stable object for extended time.

ii. Seeks light pressure
Seeking may take the form of participating in or requesting action. Examples of light pressure include drawing scarves across the skin, scratching with fingernails on skin, or requesting tickling.

iii. Tolerates firm pressure
Client participates in activities involving firm pressure without distress or resistance. Examples of firm pressure include rolling a cabasa on the body or placing therapist's hands on the body.

iv. Tolerates light pressure
Client participates in activities involving light pressure without distress or resistance. Examples of light pressure include drawing scarves across the skin or playing windchimes.

SKILL DEFINITIONS – SENSORY SKILLS

v. Tolerates lightweight manipulatives

Client participates in activities involving lightweight objects which must be manipulated with hands without distress or resistance. Examples of lightweight manipulatives include egg shakers, scarves, rattles, and mallets.

vi. Tolerates putting mouthpiece to lips

Client places mouthpiece of instrument to lips without resistance or distress. Ability to tolerate may differ according to material of mouthpiece (i.e., wood, plastic, metal).

vii. Demonstrates ability to begin/stop tactile activity

Client participates in and is able to stop tactile activities when cued without perseveration, resistance, or distress.

viii. Demonstrates awareness of or attends to tactile input

Client may demonstrate awareness by verbally referencing input or making observable change in eye gaze, affect, or body posture. Attention may be demonstrated by acting upon input received.

ix. Remains physically open when instrument presented

Client does not close hands, cross legs, fold arms, etc., upon presentation of instrument.

x. Sustains grasp of instrument or mallet for four seconds or more

Client holds instrument or mallet for a minimum of four seconds.

xi. Uses open hand on instruments

Client uses palm of hand to play drum, cabasa, or other instrument.

C. Proprioceptive

General definition. Proprioceptive input is information received from musculo/skeletal systems and senses which supply information as to awareness of body in space. Examples of activities which create proprioceptive input may include standing, running, pushing, pulling, and extension of arms or legs.

i. Seeks proprioceptive input

Seeking may take the form of participating in or requesting action.

ii. Tolerates proprioceptive input
Client participates in activities involving proprioceptive input without distress or resistance.

iii. Demonstrates ability to begin/stop proprioceptive activity
Client participates in and is able to stop proprioceptive activities when cued without perseveration, resistance, or distress.

iv. Integrates proprioceptive tasks into activities
Client participates in musical activities that involve proprioceptive input such as falling down in "Ring Around the Rosy," and movement of body parts in "The Hokey Pokey."

D. Vestibular

General definition. The vestibular system's function is to orient the head in space (balance). Examples of activities that affect the vestibular system include rocking, spinning, jumping, twisting, and swinging arms from side to side across the midline.

i. Seeks vestibular input
Seeking may take the form of participating in or requesting action.

ii. Tolerates vestibular input
Client participates in activities involving vestibular input without distress or resistance.

iii. Demonstrates ability to begin/stop vestibular activity
Client participates in and is able to stop vestibular activities when cued, without perseveration, resistance, or distress.

iv. Demonstrates ability to return to task after vestibular distraction with prompts
Client returns to presented activity after unrelated vestibular stimulation such as rocking or jumping. Prompts may include verbal, visual, physical, or musical.

v. Demonstrates ability to return to task after vestibular distraction without prompts
Client returns to presented activity after unrelated vestibular stimulation such as rocking or jumping.

E. Visual

General definition. Visual input is any information seen or able to be seen by the eye.

i. Seeks visual input

Seeking may take the form of participating in or requesting action. Examples may include light gazing, flapping hands in front of eyes, or manipulation of environment for visual stimulation (lining up of objects or precise placement of objects).

ii. Tolerates visual input

Client participates in activities involving visual input without distress or resistance. Examples include viewing pictures or colors, use of a light source, or arranging objects.

iii. Demonstrates ability to begin/stop visual activity

Client participates in and is able to stop visual activities when cued, without perseveration, resistance, or distress.

iv. Demonstrates ability to return to task after visual distraction with prompts

Client returns to presented activity after unrelated visual stimulation such as movements in periphery. Prompts may include verbal, visual, physical, or musical.

v. Demonstrates awareness of or attends to visual input

Client may demonstrate awareness by verbally referencing input or making observable change in eye gaze, affect, or body posture. Attention may be demonstrated by acting upon input received.

vi. Maintains gaze of object or person for appropriate length

Client visually references object or person without visual perseveration or visual avoidance.

vii. Demonstrates ability to return to task after visual distraction without prompts

Client returns to presented activity after unrelated visual stimulation such as movements in periphery.

F. Auditory

General definition. Auditory input is any and all sounds.

i. Seeks auditory input

Examples of seeking auditory input may include holding instrument close to ears, turning up volume, creating loud dynamics (vocally or instrumentally), or perseveration on a certain sound (scratching or squeaking).

ii. Demonstrates awareness of sound vs. silence

Client demonstrates observable or musical response to sound vs. silence, such as changes in eye gaze, affect, or body movement.

iii. Tolerates auditory input

Client participates in activities involving auditory input without distress or resistance.

iv. Tolerates a variety of sounds

Client participates in activities involving a variety of sounds without distress or resistance. Examples may include piano and drum, voice and cabasa, or ocean drum and recorder.

v. Demonstrates ability to begin/stop auditory activity

Client participates in and is able to stop auditory activities when cued without perseveration, resistance, or distress.

vi. Demonstrates awareness of or attends to auditory input

Client may demonstrate awareness by verbally referencing input or making observable change in eye gaze, affect, or body posture. Attention may be demonstrated by acting upon input received.

vii. Demonstrates ability to return to task after auditory distraction with prompts

Client returns to presented activity after unrelated auditory stimulation such as environmental noises. Prompts may include verbal, visual, physical, or musical.

viii. Demonstrates ability to return to task after auditory distraction without prompts

Client returns to presented activity after unrelated auditory stimulation such as environmental noises.

Receptive communication/auditory perception (RC)

A. Fundamentals

i. Demonstrates awareness of sound vs. silence

Client demonstrates observable response to sound vs. silence, such as changes in eye gaze, affect, respiration, body movement, etc.

ii. Turns head to sound source

Client demonstrates localization behavior by turning his/her head towards a sound source within 2 seconds of sound production.

iii. Localizes eye gaze to sound source

Client demonstrates localization behavior by shifting eye gaze towards a sound source within 2 seconds of sound production.

iv. Discriminates between two different sounds

Client indicates through verbal or nonverbal communication differentiation of two distinct sounds. Examples are varied actions in response to drum vs. cymbal, or naming instrument from auditory cues only.

v. Imitates simple musical motif

Client reproduces a musical motif of two or more notes immediately after modeling.

B. Direction following

i. Follows one-step verbal direction

Client performs a one-step verbal direction (e.g., "Hold this mallet.") on command. Does not include directions in which a choice must be made such as "Choose an instrument."

ii. Follows two-step verbal direction

Client takes action when directed by therapist with sung or spoken direction. Examples of two-step verbal directions are "Sit down and play the cabasa," or "March to the table and play the drum." Does not include directions in which a choice must be made such as "Sit down and choose an instrument."

iii. Follows simple musical cues

Client performs actions in response to simple musical cues (e.g., start/stop, call and response).

C. Musical changes

i. Demonstrates awareness of gross tempo changes

Client verbally references or makes observable changes in eye gaze, affect, respiration, body movement, etc., in response to gross tempo change (e.g., vivace to largo).

ii. Demonstrates awareness of gross pitch changes

Client verbally references or makes observable changes in eye gaze, affect, respiration, body movement, etc., in response to gross pitch change of an octave or more.

iii. Demonstrates awareness of gross dynamic changes

Client verbally references or makes observable changes in eye gaze, affect, respiration, body movement, etc., in response to gross dynamic change (e.g., piano to forte).

iv. Demonstrates awareness of meter changes

Client verbally references or makes observable changes in eye gaze, affect, respiration, body movement, etc., in response to meter change (e.g., 3/4 to 4/4).

v. Demonstrates awareness of changes in intensity/mood

Client verbally references or makes observable changes in eye gaze, affect, respiration, body movement, etc., in response to changes in intensity or mood (e.g., somber to playful).

vi. Plays melodically in tonality of improvisation

Client plays a melody in the tonality (e.g., major, minor, pentatonic, or modal) of the therapist's improvisation.

vii. Plays in appropriate key without prompting
Client plays a melody, chords, or combination thereof in the tonality (e.g., major, minor, pentatonic, or modal) of the therapist's improvisation without prompts.

D. Singing/vocalizing

i. Vocalizes in response to aural stimuli
Client produces vocalizations when he/she hears environmental noise, talking, singing, and/or musical instruments in the clinical setting; vocalizations may occur intermittently or continuously in response to aural stimuli in the environment.

ii. Vocalizes in response to therapist speaking
Client produces vocalizations during or immediately after the therapist speaks.

iii. Vocalizes in response to therapist singing
Client produces vocalizations during or immediately after the therapist sings.

iv. Vocalizes in response to un-pitched instruments
Client produces vocalizations during or immediately after un-pitched instruments such as drums and hand percussion are played.

v. Vocalizes in response to pitched instruments
Client produces vocalizations during or immediately after pitched instruments such as piano or xylophone are played.

vi. Vocalizes in response to a particular musical style/idiom
Client produces vocalizations during or immediately after a particular musical style, mode, or scale is played.

vii. Unconscious vocalizations in tonality
Client's vocalizations appear to be unintended or involuntary, yet reflect the tonality of the music being played (e.g., major, minor, pentatonic, or modal).

viii. Sings in key with therapist
Client sings in the key of the therapist and/or the musical accompaniment being played.

ix. Vocalizes in provided musical pause
Client vocalizes when cued by pause in music, such as completing a known song phrase or finishing a bar of rhythmic measure.

x. Imitates descending musical interval greater than M2
Client reproduces melodically descending interval of more than major 2nd immediately after modeling.

xi. Imitates ascending musical interval greater than M2
Client reproduces melodically ascending interval of more than major 2nd immediately after modeling.

xii. Sings pitched melody accurately
Client sings the correct pitches of a melody.

xiii. Imitates descending step-wise musical motifs
Client reproduces a melodically descending motif of no more than major 2nd intervals immediately after modeling.

xiv. Imitates ascending step-wise musical motifs
Client reproduces a melodically ascending motif of no more than major 2nd intervals immediately after modeling.

E. Rhythm

i. Plays in tempo of therapist 1–4 measures
Client plays an instrument matching therapist's tempo for a minimum of one measure.

ii. Imitates simple rhythmic pattern
Client reproduces a rhythmic pattern of one measure in duple or triple meter using quarter and eighth note values immediately after modeling.

iii. Imitates intermediate rhythmic pattern
Client reproduces a rhythmic pattern of one measure in duple or triple meter using quarter and eighth note values, triplets, and dotted quarters immediately after modeling.

Expressive communication (EC)

General definition. Expressive communication includes eye contact, facial expression, gesture, sign, augmentative or alternative communication systems, vocalization, or verbalization.

A. Fundamentals

i. Attempts to communicate

Client uses eye contact, facial expression, gesture, sign, vocalization, or verbalization to send a message.

ii. Communicates without frustration

Client is able to produce verbal or nonverbal communication without observable distress.

iii. Communicates needs and desires

Client uses verbal or nonverbal communication to accurately express needs and desires.

iv. Communicates ideas and concepts

Client uses verbal or nonverbal communication to express thoughts, ideas, concepts, and knowledge that extend beyond the scope of needs and desires.

v. Communicates emotional content or idea development

Client can effectively express emotions of self and others and develop ideas beyond his/her basic concept level.

B. Non-vocal communication

General definition. Non-vocal communication includes eye contact, facial expression, gesture, sign, augmentative or alternative communication systems.

i. Leads or moves therapist as means of communication

Client purposefully manipulates the therapist's body or body parts to express a need, desire, or concept.

ii. Gestures

Client moves his/her body or body parts to communicate a need, desire, or concept.

iii. Combines gesture with leading/moving of therapist

Client uses a more complex nonverbal means of communicating by combining gesture and moving or leading the therapist.

iv. Combines gesture with vocalization

Client uses a more complex means of communicating by simultaneously or subsequently gesturing and vocalizing.

C. Vocalizations

General definition. Vocalizations include words and/or vocal sounds that are not recognizable to the examiner as words or word approximations. Examples include babble, nonsense sounds, or humming.

i. Vocalizations are of clear tonal quality

Client produces vocalizations without hoarseness, breathiness, or strain.

ii. Vocalizations are of appropriate volume

Client produces vocalizations at a volume appropriate to/within the action, environment, or activity.

iii. Vocalizations are in moderate pitch range

Client produces vocalizations at a pitch range appropriate to/within the action, environment, or activity.

iv. Vocalizations are of phrase length

Client produces vocalizations equivalent in duration to an utterance of 2–3 words.

v. Vocalizations are of sentence length

Client produces vocalizations equivalent in duration to an utterance of 3 or more words.

D. Spontaneous vocalizations

General definition. Spontaneous vocalizations are words and/or vocal sounds that are independently produced by the client without visual, verbal, or physical prompting.

i. Vocalizes with therapist

Client produces vocalizations simultaneously with the therapist without prompting.

ii. Vocalizations are of non-imitative type

Client produces vocalizations that differ in aspects of modeled pitch, melody, and/or rhythm from what was presented by the therapist immediately prior to the vocalization.

iii. Vocalizations are purposefully imitative

Client produces vocalizations that share a majority of characteristics of modeled pitch, melody, and/or rhythm with what was presented by the therapist immediately previous to the vocalization.

E. Verbalizations

General definition. Verbalizations are spoken or sung word or word approximations. Verbalizations may include jargon containing words, echolalia, or scripted content.

i. Verbalizations are intelligible

Client produces words, phrases, or sentences that can be comprehended fully by the therapist.

ii. Verbalizes single words

Client produces verbalizations that are at least one word in length. Examples include "No," "Bye," "Play."

iii. Verbalizations are of phrase length

Client produces verbalizations that are approximately 2–3 words in length and may or may not constitute a grammatically complete sentence.

iv. Verbalizations are of sentence length

Client produces verbalizations that are approximately 3–6 words in length and may or may not constitute a grammatically complete sentence.

F. Relational communication

General definition. Relational communications are those verbal or nonverbal communications which take place in an interactive manner with another individual.

i. Answers closed (yes/no) questions

Client indicates a "yes" or "no" answer to a closed question using verbal or nonverbal communication.

ii. Answers binary questions

Client indicates one answer using verbal or nonverbal communication when presented with two choices.

iii. Participates in simple reciprocal conversation

Client takes part in simple conversation regarding needs, desires, and activities of daily living using verbal or nonverbal communication.

iv. Initiates conversation appropriate to situation

Client starts a conversation by asking a question or making a comment about a topic appropriate to the time, place, or circumstance using verbal or nonverbal communication.

v. Asks questions appropriately

Client asks questions purposefully without disruption, interruption, echolalia, or perseveration.

vi. Answers open questions

Client answers complex questions that require more than a "yes," "no," or short (1–2 word) answer using verbal or nonverbal communication.

G. *Vocal idiosyncrasies*

General definition. Vocal idiosyncrasies are peculiarities in a client's speech.

i. Vocalizations contain inflectional babble/jargon

Client produces vocalizations that contain strings of nonsense sounds and syllables that have adult-like inflection (inflectional babble) or contain scripted phrases (jargon).

ii. Vocalizations are echolalic

Client produces vocalizations that echo what he/she has heard either immediately prior to the vocalization or at some time prior to the session.

iii. Vocalizations are unconscious

Client's vocalizations appear to be unintended or involuntary.

iv. Vocalizations are delayed

Client produces vocalizations more than 5 seconds after the presentation of stimuli to which he/she is responding.

v. Vocalizations are clipped or of irregular meter

Client produces vocalizations that deviate from the rate, flow, or rhythm of typical speech or vocalization.

vi. Vocalizations are scripted

Client produces vocalizations that are exact imitations of previously heard material. Examples are repeating dialogue from media, or perseveration on lyrical content. Does not require imitation of inflection or speaking tone.

Cognitive skills (COG)

A. Fundamentals

i. Sustains activity-length attention span

Client attends to activity from beginning to end; i.e., remains in proximity, does not demonstrate distraction, or disrupt activity. Does not include activities that extend beyond typical and reasonable limits for age as judged by music therapist.

ii. Looks for hidden or dropped object

Client demonstrates understanding of object permanence by looking for object or instrument which has been presented to client and then hidden or dropped. Client may also demonstrate understanding of object permanence by asking for object or instrument used previously which is not currently in sight or referring to/requesting object, instrument, or person outside of room.

iii. Demonstrates understanding of rules and structures

Client follows directions, begins, and stops activities as directed and uses instruments for intended or described use.

B. Decision making

i. Answers closed (yes/no) questions

Client indicates a "yes" or "no" answer to a closed question using verbal or nonverbal communication.

ii. Makes choice between two presented concrete options

Client indicates a preference between two presented concrete options such as drum or piano through verbal or nonverbal communication. Presentation of options may take the form of verbal, visual, or auditory cues.

iii. Makes choice between three presented concrete options

Client indicates a preference between three presented concrete options such as drum, piano, or guitar through verbal or nonverbal communication. Presentation of options may take the form of verbal, visual, or auditory cues.

iv. Answers abstract binary questions

Client indicates one answer using verbal or nonverbal communication when presented with two abstract choices. Examples are "Are you feeling happy or sad?" or "Do you want slow or fast music?"

v. Makes choice without prompting

When presented with a choice, client indicates preference through verbal or nonverbal communication without further prompting by music therapist.

C. Direction following

i. Follows one-step verbal direction

Client performs a one-step verbal direction (e.g., "Hold this mallet.") on command. Does not include directions in which a choice must be made such as "Choose an instrument."

ii. Follows two-step verbal direction

Client takes action when directed by therapist with sung or spoken direction. Examples of two-step verbal directions are "Sit down and play the cabasa," or "March to the table and play the drum." Does not include directions in which a choice must be made such as "Sit down and choose an instrument."

iii. Follows simple musical cues

Client performs actions in response to simple musical cues (e.g., start/stop, call and response).

D. Short-term recall/sequencing

i. Recalls new information within activity

Client demonstrates recall of new information presented within the activity, such as repeating words in a song, sequencing instruments in the correct order, or playing presented rhythmic patterns. Echolalia is acceptable as it does demonstrate short-term recall.

ii. Sequences two objects within activity

Client plays two differing instruments in succession and in the same order as previously presented by therapist.

iii. Sequences three objects within activity

Client plays three differing instruments in succession and in the same order as previously presented by therapist.

E. Long-term recall

Note: This section is assessed only if the client is seen for more than one session.

i. Recalls therapist's name

Client verbally or nonverbally communicates therapist's name with or without cueing but not imitatively.

ii. Recalls name of instrument

Client identifies instrument presented in previous session by verbally or nonverbally communicating name or selecting correct instrument when named by therapist.

iii. Recalls function of instruments

Client demonstrates knowledge of instrument presented in previous session by playing in manner consistent with previous experience.

iv. Demonstrates awareness of MT routine

Client enters room and takes place at area typically used for greeting song or interaction with minimal prompting; transitions between activities without distress or refusal; and leaves room after goodbye song or interaction.

v. Requests previously presented activities/songs

Client, through verbal or nonverbal communication, indicates a desire to repeat activities or songs presented in previous music therapy session. Perseveration is acceptable as it does demonstrate long-term recall.

vi. Sings correct lyrics without visual/aural cues

Client sings correct words to song presented in previous music therapy session without verbal or written cues. Musical cues (such as accompaniment and melody) are acceptable. Does not imply client must sing correct melody or rhythm.

vii. Plays simple accompaniment without visual/aural cues

Client plays chords of a song presented in a previous music therapy session without verbal or written cues. Must consist of two or more chords for at least two measures with no pulse or rhythm required. Permissable for therapist to sing/play with client.

viii. Plays intermediate accompaniment without visual/aural cues

Client plays chords of a song presented in a previous music therapy session without verbal or written cues. Must consist of four or more chords for at least four measures with no pulse or rhythm required. Permissable for therapist to sing/play with client.

ix. Plays advanced accompaniment without visual/aural cues

Client plays chords of a song presented in a previous music therapy session without verbal or written cues. Must consist of four or more chords for at least four measures with pulse and rhythm required. Permissable for therapist to sing/play with client.

F. Academics

i. Matches three colors

Client correctly chooses three primary colors to correspond with presented same colors. Colors may be presented in the form of color cue cards, colored scarves, or solid colored instruments.

ii. Matches three symbols

Client correctly chooses three pictures to correspond with presented same objects or pictures, such as PECS, clipart, photographs. Symbols must be high-quality, clearly indicated representations of objects.

iii. Identifies three colors

Client indicates, through verbal or nonverbal communication, the names of three primary colors (i.e., blue, red, yellow, green). Indication may take the form of pointing to written word, stating word, or selecting correct color from verbal or written cue.

iv. Cued by written symbol to complete or begin task

Client responds to written symbol by starting or stopping task when cued. Written symbols are any written letter, picture, word, or color.

v. Reads simple chord chart

Client correctly identifies a minimum of two chords from a simple chord chart. A simple chord chart is defined as written letters A–G without sharps or flats. Identification may take the form of verbally stating or playing the chords on an instrument without letter names. If playing, no pulse or rhythm required; assessment of reading skills only.

vi. Demonstrates understanding of number concepts 1–6

Client indicates, through verbal or nonverbal communication, the ability to understand and use numbers 1–6 as a quantifying measure. Indication may take the form of pointing to the correct number to indicate number of objects or playing correct number of beats from verbal or visual cue. Not defined as matching number symbols as in case of playing correct note on labeled xylophone from verbal number cue.

vii. Identifies letters A–G

Client indicates, through verbal or nonverbal communication, the names of letters A–G from written alphabet cues. Indication may take the form of pointing to correct letter, stating letter from visual cue, or playing correct labeled note on xylophone from verbal cue. Not defined as matching letter symbols as in case of playing correct note on labeled xylophone from written alphabet cue.

viii. Plays simple accompaniment using chord chart

Client plays correct chords on any harmonic instrument from standard written chord chart consisting of two or more chords and at least two measures. No pulse or rhythm required. Simple chord chart is defined as written letters A–G without sharps or flats.

ix. Plays simple melody using written letter cues

Client plays correct notes on melodic instrument from written note names. Simple melody is defined as written letters A–G without sharps or flats and with no more than four notes, maximum two measures. No pulse or rhythm required.

x. Reads lyrics

Client verbally states or sings correct words from written lyrics of newly presented children's song, folk song, or other age-appropriate material. Does not include activities that extend beyond typical and reasonable limits for age as judged by music therapist.

xi. Demonstrates ability to write lyrics

Client is able to write lyrics of known or unique song in a readable format.

xii. Reads treble clef notation

Client correctly states names of or performs notes from middle C to F within the treble clef staff, not including upper ledger lines, using IMTAP Music Sample Hiv/Hv.

xiii. Reads bass clef notation

Client correctly states names of notes or performs notes from G to middle C within the bass clef staff, not including lower ledger lines, using IMTAP Music Sample Hvi/Hvii.

xiv. Reads and plays bass and treble clef together

Client correctly performs notes from within the grand staff using IMTAP Music Sample Hix.

xv. Transcribes musical ideas using symbols or notation

Client uses written symbols or musical notation to record or communicate rhythmic or melodic idea, such as letter names, arrows, melodic contours, shapes, or colors.

Emotional skills (EMO)

A. Fundamentals

i. Demonstrates range of affect

Client shows variety in facial expression, body language, and vocal tone. Client does not demonstrate flat or restricted affect.

ii. Demonstrates appropriate affect

Client demonstrates facial expressions, body language, and vocal tone which communicate emotions appropriate to the circumstances. Does not infer that client must only exhibit positive emotions.

B. Differentiation/expression

i. Expresses emotions appropriate to circumstances

Client conveys feelings or mood through verbal, nonverbal, or musical means congruent to situation.

ii. Expresses emotions using instruments

Client conveys feelings or mood using musical components such as rhythm, timbre, or dynamics.

iii. Expresses emotions verbally

Client conveys feelings or mood using verbal means.

iv. Demonstrates emotional sensitivity to musical components

Client demonstrates observable change in eye gaze, affect, respiration, body movement, etc., in response to overt emotional components of music such as mode, key, tempo, or dynamic.

C. Regulation

i. Tolerates MT situation without distress

Client is able to be present in music therapy situation without exhibiting clear signs of upset or disturbance such as crying, moaning, or screaming.

ii. Calms with support
Client is able to reduce exhibited distress in response to musical, verbal, or physical support from therapist.

iii. Tolerates transitions
Client changes activities without distress or refusal.

iv. Self-regulates within one activity
Regulation is the absence of apparent distress, self-stimulation, or distracting behaviors.

v. Emotional states fluctuate appropriately
Client does not exhibit rapid mood swings or emotional changes unrelated to present circumstance.

vi. Remains regulated when limits are set
Client is able to remain regulated when procedures, rules, or parameters are presented by therapist. Regulation is the absence of apparent distress, self-stimulation, or distracting behaviors.

D. Self-awareness

i. Demonstrates recognition of emotional states
Recognition of emotional states could be demonstrated through client verbally identifying or labeling own or others' emotional states; visually selecting image corresponding to emotional state; or playing music related to emotional state.

ii. Demonstrates ability to explore emotional states
Exploration of emotional states could be demonstrated through client verbally discussing own or others' emotional state; musical compositions based on emotional ideas; or lyric analysis of emotional components.

iii. Demonstrates ability to discuss emotional states
Client demonstrates ability to discuss own or others' emotional states verbally or using alternative communication.

iv. Initiates emotional content appropriately

When given an opportunity, client initiates musical exploration or verbal discussion of emotional content. Does not include perseveration on emotional topics to exclusion or disruption of other activities.

v. Demonstrates desire to better oneself or life circumstance

Client initiates verbal discussion or lyrical composition which identifies desired changes in life or life situation, such as learning a self-help skill, or improving classroom participation.

Social skills (SOC)

A. Fundamentals

i. Responds to own name

Client demonstrates reaction to use of own name in conversation or music. Reactions may include looking toward therapist, stopping current action, redirecting attention, or verbally responding.

ii. Demonstrates awareness of therapist

Client looks toward therapist for cueing, verbally addresses therapist, or follows musical cues provided by therapist.

iii. Demonstrates interest in presented activities

Interest may be demonstrated by client reaching toward or playing presented instruments; asking for certain activities or songs; or showing expectant affect while participating.

iv. Demonstrates joint attention

Client uses verbal or nonverbal communication, eye contact, and/or gesture for the social purpose of sharing experiences and information.

v. Interacts appropriately with therapist

Client participates in a manner free of verbal abuse or physical harm directed towards the therapist.

vi. Uses socially appropriate greeting

Examples of socially appropriate greetings are "Hello," "Hi," or "How are you?" Greeting may take the form of gesture but may not include jargon or out-of-context greetings.

vii. Uses socially appropriate goodbye

Examples of socially appropriate goodbyes are "Bye," "Goodbye," or "See you later." Greeting may take the form of gesture but may not include jargon or out-of-context greetings.

viii. Uses socially appropriate eye contact

Client makes eye contact that is of appropriate length (i.e., more than fleeting but not of perseverative nature).

ix. Socially references others

Client looks to therapist for affirmation or to assess response before, during, or after activity.

x. Demonstrates understanding of rules and structures

Client follows directions, begins, and stops activities as directed and uses instruments for intended or described use.

xi. Demonstrates awareness of appropriate physical space

Client adjusts proximity to therapist based on context of activity. Examples may include sitting closely on piano bench and moving away during marching activity.

xii. Demonstrates confidence in MT situation

Client participates in activities without extensive encouragement or verbal support.

B. *Participation*

i. Enters room with minimal prompting

Client enters therapy room with less than three prompts or cues.

ii. Remains in room for duration of session

Client remains in therapy room from beginning to end of session.

iii. Attempts new tasks when given opportunity

Client participates in unfamiliar activities or experiences when introduced by therapist.

iv. Initiates new activity when given opportunity

Client changes activity independently after close of previous activity, during transition, or when prompted by therapist. Client may reach towards new instrument, request, or begin new activity.

v. Tolerates transitions

Client changes activities without distress or refusal.

vi. Participates in structured activities

Client participates in activity with clearly defined procedures, rules, or parameters, such as "Hokey Pokey" or "Freeze Dance."

vii. Is flexible in developing activities

Client participates in extension and development of activities without distress or refusal.

viii. Extends activities appropriately

Client extends activities without perseveration or refusal to end activity.

ix. Works towards identified goals in session

Client makes focused efforts to complete personal goals as identified in session, such as learning a song on guitar or piano, or mastering a rhythmic pattern.

C. Turn-taking

i. Anticipates own turn

Client demonstrates anticipation of turn through immediately taking turn at appropriate time, keeping visual contact, or filling in responses during anticipatory response activity.

ii. Waits for turn

Client allows therapist to complete turn before playing or performing action during established turn-taking activity.

iii. Sustains turn-taking with prompts

Participates in turn-taking activity of four or more cycles. Prompts may be visual, verbal, physical, or musical.

iv. Requests turn when appropriate

Client verbally or by gesture requests turn. Does not include client repeatedly asking for turn to the disturbance of therapist's turns or precluding the completion of the activity.

v. Sustains turn-taking without prompts

Participates in turn-taking activity of at least four cycles. Without prompts is defined as without visual, verbal, or physical prompts. Does not include musical prompts such as cadences, repeated musical motifs, or length of rhythmic passage in turn-taking.

D. Attention

i. Sustains activity-length attention span

Client attends to activity from beginning to end; i.e., remains in proximity, does not demonstrate distraction, or disrupt activity. Does not include activities that extend beyond typical and reasonable limits for age as judged by MT.

ii. Demonstrates sustained attention to therapist

Client attends to the therapist for one minute or more without self-stimulation, perserveration, or off-task behavior. Client may, during this time, briefly break eye gaze.

iii. Returns to activity after distraction with prompts

Distraction may be defined as any aural, visual, or tactile input unrelated to the activity. Prompts may include verbal, visual, musical, or physical prompts.

iv. Returns to activity after distraction without prompts

Distraction may be defined as any aural, visual, or tactile input unrelated to the activity.

E. Direction following

i. Follows one-step verbal direction

Client performs a one-step verbal direction, such as "Hold this mallet," on command. Does not include directions in which a choice must be made, such as "Choose an instrument."

ii. Follows two-step verbal direction

Client takes action when directed by therapist with sung or spoken direction. Examples of two-step verbal directions are "Sit down and play the cabasa," or "March to the table and play the drum." Does not include directions in which a choice must be made, such as "Sit down and choose an instrument."

iii. Follows simple musical cues

Client takes action when musically directed by therapist. Musical cues may include start/stop, call and response, cadence, or unfinished melodic phrase.

F. Relationship skills

i. Tolerates direct interaction

Client does not exhibit distress or resistance when sung, played, or talked to.

ii. Tolerates redirection

Client is able to be redirected without demonstrating resistance or distress.

iii. Tolerates musical contact

Client is able to listen to and/or participate in music without demonstrating resistance or distress.

iv. Plays in parallel with therapist

Client plays music simultaneously with therapist. Does not require client to play in tempo, rhythm, correct key, or otherwise adapt to therapist's music.

v. Plays in imitation of therapist

Client imitates musical ideas of therapist. Imitation can be rhythmical, melodic, in mood, or physical.

vi. Sustains musical interaction
Client plays or sings music with therapist for one minute or more.

vii. Sustains two-way communication
Client demonstrates ability to participate in communication with therapist for one minute or more. Communication may take the form of verbal discussion, gesture, sign, or adaptive communication devices.

viii. Works cooperatively with therapist
Client demonstrates ability to work with therapist towards a common goal, such as maintaining a steady pulse while therapist plays melody, or planning the session with the therapist.

ix. Demonstrates flexibility in interactive musical play
Client is able to adapt to changes without distress or resistance within improvised, unstructured, musical exploration of sounds, movements, instruments, props, or voice with therapist. Examples are vocal glissandos, slide whistle play, and xylophone exploration.

x. Demonstrates flexibility within familiar interactive structure
Client is able to adapt to changes without distress or resistance while participating in familiar activity with therapist, such as changing words to a known song, changing rules to a musical game, or substituting instruments within a musical activity.

xi. Can assume leadership role in activity
Client demonstrates ability to direct or lead interaction or activity.

xii. Moves between independent and interdependent skills
Client demonstrates ability to transition between independent and interactive roles in an activity. Client does not exhibit resistance or distress in either independent or interdependent work.

xiii. Able to explore external social relationships
External social relationships are defined as relationships which occur outside of the music therapy session, such as relationships with friends or family members. Exploration may take the form of discussion or musical composition.

Musicality (MUS)

A. Fundamentals

i. Is alerted by music

Client demonstrates awareness of music by observable changes in eye gaze, affect, respiration, body movement, etc.

ii. Expresses enjoyment of music

Client displays pleasure during or after presentation of music as observed by facial expression, gesture, body movement, sign, vocalization, or verbalization. Examples may include smiling, laughing, tapping feet, or dancing.

iii. Indicates desire to play/touch instruments

Client demonstrates desire by reaching for instrument, directing eye gaze toward instrument, or vocalization/verbalization.

iv. Plays instrument when presented

Client plays instrument when offered by therapist.

v. Explores instruments

Client explores sound, timbre, range, shape, or positioning of instrument.

vi. Vocalizes in response to music

Client produces vocalizations during or after presentation of music. Vocalizations are defined as any sound produced by the organs of speech.

vii. Moves rhythmically in response to music

Client moves in a regular, steady tempo; e.g., rocks, walks, dances, sways, jumps, snaps, nods, during or immediately after presentation of music. Does not require client to match tempo of music.

viii. Plays instruments spontaneously

Client independently plays instrument without visual, verbal, or physical prompting. Musical stimuli may be present.

ix. Sings spontaneously
Client independently sings without visual, verbal, or physical prompting. Musical stimuli may be present.

x. Responds to musical cue
Client produces an observable behavior, such as changes in eye gaze, affect, respiration, body movement, etc., during or after presentation of musical cue. Musical cues may include start/stop, call and response, cadence, or unfinished melodic phrase.

xi. Engages in interactive musical play
Client participates in improvised, unstructured, musical exploration of sounds, movements, instruments, props, or voice with therapist. Examples are vocal glissandos, slide whistle play, and xylophone exploration.

xii. Regulates with musical support
When client is deregulating (e.g., exhibiting distress, leaving area, displaying off-task behavior), client is able to return to activity, attend to activity, or cease to exhibit distress in response to musical assistance, such as musical cue, familiar song, ISO Principle, or change of musical element.

B. Tempo

i. Tolerates changing tempo
Client does not cease playing, perseverate, or exhibit distress when the tempo of a song, activity, or improvisation is altered.

ii. Demonstrates awareness of gross tempo changes
Client verbally references or makes observable changes in eye gaze, affect, respiration, body movement, etc., in response to gross tempo change (e.g., vivace to largo).

iii. Unconscious body movement in tempo
Client demonstrates unintended or involuntary movement in tempo of music.

iv. Conscious body movement in tempo
Client demonstrates intended or voluntary movement in tempo of music.

v. Plays in own tempo 1–4 measures
Client independently plays instrument at own preferred tempo for 1–4 measures.

vi. Plays in tempo of therapist 1–4 measures
Client plays instrument matching the same tempo as the therapist for 1–4 measures.

vii. Initiates tempo changes
Client demonstrates, signs, or verbally indicates a different tempo from current tempo.

viii. Adapts playing to match tempo changes
Client demonstrates ability to change tempo from musical cue alone.

ix. Adapts playing to follow accelerando
Client demonstrates ability to increase speed of playing in response to gradually faster tempo.

x. Sustains playing in own tempo interactively
Client independently plays instrument at own preferred tempo for more than four measures with therapist.

xi. Sustains playing in tempo of therapist interactively
Client plays instrument matching the same tempo as the therapist for more than four measures.

xii. Plays multiples of basic beat
Client plays regular subdivisions of the presented pulse, such as eighths, triplets, dotted eighths.

xiii. Adapts playing to follow ritardando
Client demonstrates ability to decrease speed of playing in response to gradually slower tempo.

C. Rhythm

i. Imitates simple rhythmic pattern
Client reproduces a rhythmic pattern of one measure in duple or triple meter using quarter and eighth note values immediately after modeling, such as a simple name pattern starting on the upbeat or first beat of the bar.

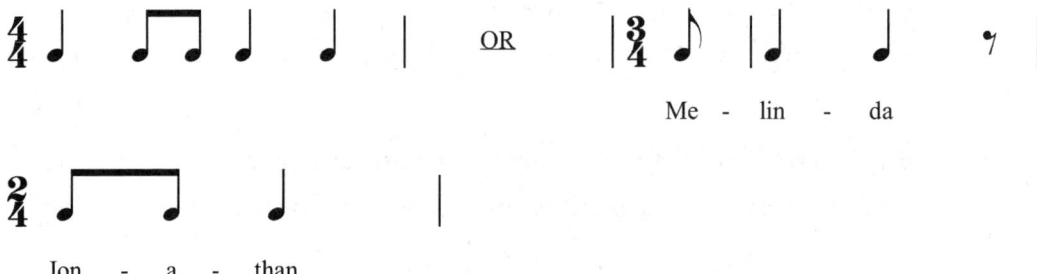

Me - lin - da

Jon - a - than

ii. Imitates intermediate rhythmic pattern
Client reproduces a rhythmic pattern of one measure in duple or triple meter using quarter and eighth note values, triplets, and dotted quarters immediately after modeling.

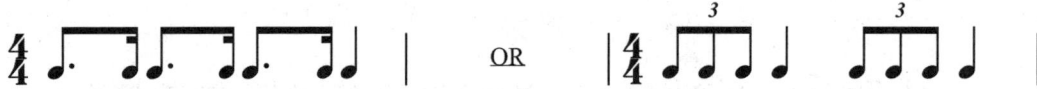

iii. Beats rhythmic pattern of melody or words
Client translates sung or spoken pattern in rhythmic form on instrument.

iv. Sustains imitation of varying rhythmic patterns
Client repeats differing rhythmic patterns as presented by therapist for four or more consecutive turns.

v. Changes rhythmic pattern in response to music
Client independently alters rhythmic pattern during musical interaction.

SKILL DEFINITIONS – MUSICALITY

vi. Coordinates two differing rhythmic patterns

Client coordinates two rhythmic patterns simultaneously; i.e., plays quarter notes with left hand and half notes with right, or accents final beat in measure with second instrument.

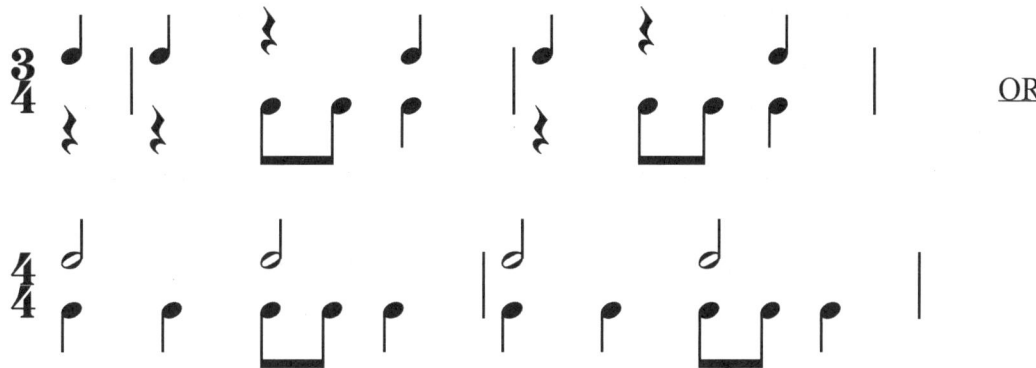

vii. Initiates differing rhythmic patterns during turn-taking

Client independently creates non-imitative rhythmic patterns during turn-taking with therapist.

viii. Initiates rhythmic structures involving multiple patterns

Client independently creates a rhythmic motif consisting of two or more rhythmic patterns played consecutively with at least one repetition of the entire motif; e.g., four quarter notes followed by a triplet combination with entire form repeated at least once.

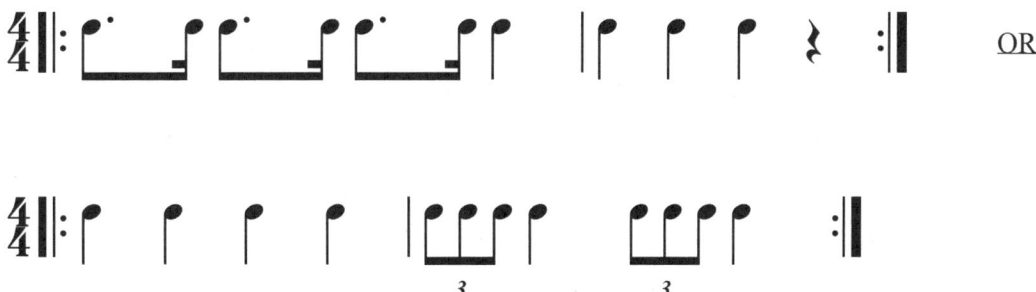

ix. Develops rhythmic structures involving multiple patterns

Client independently changes or builds upon a rhythmic motif consisting of two or more rhythmic patterns played consecutively with at least one repetition of the entire motif; e.g., four quarter notes followed by a triplet combination with entire form repeated at least once.

x. Sustains self-initiated rhythmic patterns
Client plays non-imitative rhythmic patterns for more than four measures.

xi. Adapts playing to match meter changes
Client demonstrates ability to change meter from musical cue alone.

D. Dynamics

i. Demonstrates awareness of gross dynamic changes
Client verbally references or makes observable changes in eye gaze, affect, respiration, body movement, etc., in response to gross dynamic change (e.g., piano to forte).

ii. Tolerates changing dynamic
Client does not cease playing, perseverate, or exhibit distress when the dynamic of a song, activity, or improvisation is altered.

iii. Demonstrates variety of dynamics in playing
Client demonstrates the ability to play a range of dynamics in playing.

iv. Initiates dynamic changes
Client demonstrates, signs, or verbally indicates a different dynamic from the current dynamic.

v. Follows cue to change dynamic
Client increases or decreases volume of playing in response to visual, verbal, or musical cue.

vi. Adapts playing to crescendo
Client demonstrates ability to increase volume of playing in response to gradually louder music.

vii. Adapts playing to diminuendo
Client demonstrates ability to decrease volume of playing in response to gradually quieter music.

viii. Demonstrates control of crescendo
Client demonstrates ability to gradually increase volume of playing or vocalizing.

ix. Demonstrates control of diminuendo
Client demonstrates ability to gradually decrease volume of playing or vocalizing.

x. Demonstrates expressive use of diminuendo/crescendo
Client spontaneously utilizes increase and decrease in volume during playing or vocalizing to communicate mood, emotion, or content.

E. Vocal

i. Unconscious vocalizations in tonality
Client's vocalizations appear to be unintended or involuntary, yet reflect the tonality of the music being played (e.g., major, minor, pentatonic, or modal).

ii. Vocalizes in response to particular musical style/idiom
Client produces vocalizations during or immediately after a particular musical style, mode, or scale is played.

iii. Communicative vocalizations in tonality of music
Client uses verbal or nonverbal vocalizations to communicate a need, desire, or concept which reflect the tonality of the music being played (e.g., major, minor, pentatonic, or modal).

iv. Vocalizes to complete known song phrase
Client vocalizes the final note or notes of the end of a familiar musical phrase.

v. Sings in key or tonality
Client sings in the same tonality as the song, activity, or improvisation being played.

vi. Sings pitched melody accurately
Client sings the correct pitches of a melody.

vii. Sings using sensitivity to musical components

Client responds to or initiates a variety of musical components when singing, such as phrasing, tempo, timbre of voice, dynamics, rhythmic motifs, etc.

viii. Sings in round

Client sings own part in two-part, short vocal canon.

ix. Sings harmony line

Client sings a differentiated part in the tonality which may be pitched below or above the melody.

x. Sings expressing lyric content and meaning

Client utilizes a variety of musical components when singing, such as phrasing, tempo, timbre of voice, dynamics, rhythmic motifs, etc., to communicate mood, emotion, or content of the lyrics being sung.

xi. Creates self-expressive lyrical improvisation

Client spontaneously creates an improvisation using sung words to convey an original idea, mood, or emotion.

xii. Creates and sings own song structure

Client creates and sings musical structure consisting of at least four lines with lyrical content.

F. Perfect and relative pitch

i. Seeks and matches single tones

Client plays same note as therapist in a different pitch range or on another instrument from aural input alone; e.g., therapist playing middle C on piano and client matching on unlabeled xylophone.

ii. Plays melodically in tonality of music

Client plays melodic instrument in a manner which reflects the tonality of the music being played, such as major, minor, pentatonic, or modal, from aural input alone.

iii. Identifies letter name of tone or key per aural cue

Client communicates the correct letter name of a single tone or tonal center upon hearing it played or sung by the therapist.

iv. Initiates song in original key

Client independently plays or sings a song in the same key in which it was presented at a previous point in the session.

v. Plays known melody by ear

Client independently plays known melody without written representation or visual cue.

vi. Changes key to match changing tonality

Client alters key of own playing to match the changing tonality of the music.

vii. Transposes music by ear

Client plays recognizable musical structure in a different key from originally presented within session without written notation or visual cues.

G. Creativity and development of musical ideas

i. Creates melody independently

Client arranges musical tones to create a melodic phrase of two notes or more without therapist's assistance.

ii. Improvises melody to given rhythmic pattern

Client assigns pitched tones to a pre-determined rhythmic pattern of no more than one measure in length, in either duple or triple meter, using quarter and eighth values only.

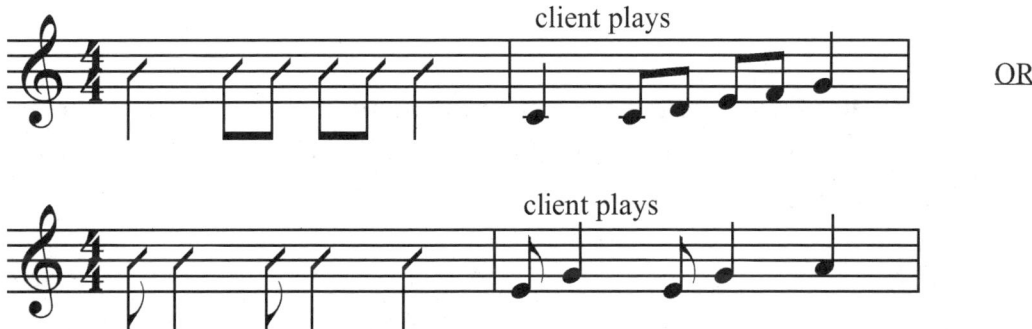

iii. Assigns differentiated instruments to given ideas or images

Client independently chooses or assigns one instrument or a series of instruments to express concepts such as a shape, a character, or a story event. For example, playing rhythm sticks to represent walking; wind chimes to represent wind; or assigning musical triangle to triangle shape; wood block to square shape; and cymbal to circular shape.

iv. Assigns differentiated musical motifs to given ideas or images

Client independently chooses or assigns a melody of two notes or more and/or a rhythmic pattern of at least one beat to express concepts such as a shape, a character, or a story event or assigning story elements to motifs played by therapist. Examples are a rhythmic motif to represent a bear walking, or glissando to represent falling.

v. Creates music to poem or story

Client arranges sounds and musical components to express content in a given poem or story.

vi. Improvises words to given rhythmic pattern

Client independently invents and performs words to match a presented rhythmic pattern.

vii. Improvises rhythmic structure

Client spontaneously invents and performs a pitched, un-pitched, or vocal rhythmic form consisting of two or more rhythmic patterns played consecutively with at least one repetition of the entire motif; e.g., four quarter notes followed by a triplet combination with entire form repeated at least once.

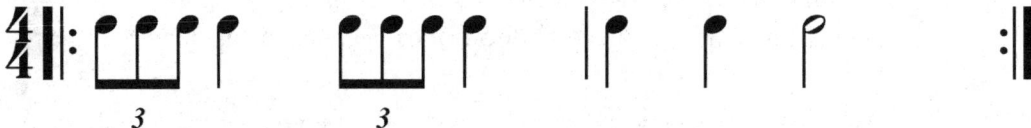

viii. Initiates phrase length musical idea in call and response

Client creates new musical motif of one or more measures during call and response activity.

ix. Creates melodic phrase with harmonic support

Client creates a melodic line of one or more measures over a presented harmonic sequence.

x. Improvises harmony

Client spontaneously invents and performs a pitched motif above or below a given melody in the correct tonality.

xi. Extends known structure through improvisation

Client participates in a familiar song and then lengthens it by spontaneously inventing and performing pitched, un-pitched, or vocal music. Client's music must differ from the familiar song but be related by tonality, rhythm, style, content, and/or mood.

xii. Creates complete song structure

Client creates and combines original lyrics and melody to form a complete song of at least one verse of at least four lines.

xiii. Transcribes musical ideas using symbols or notation

Client uses written symbols or musical notation to record or communicate rhythmic or melodic idea, such as letter names, arrows, melodic contours, shapes, or colors.

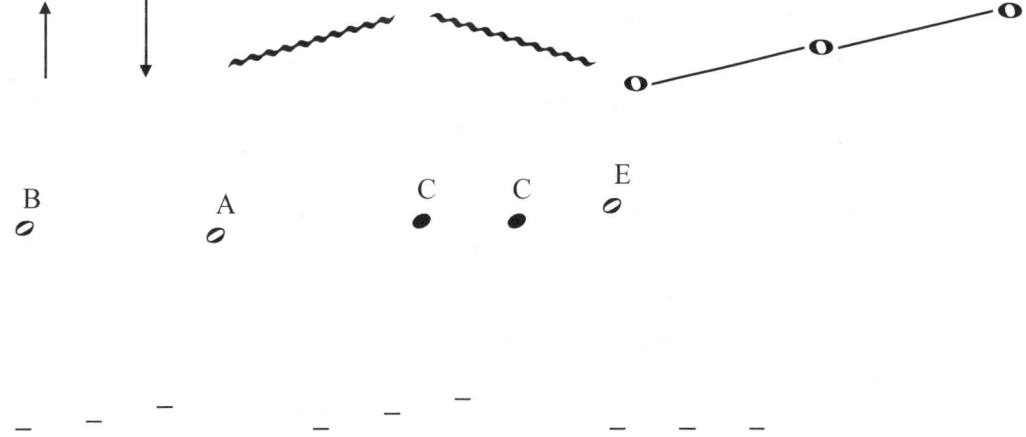

xiv. Improvises expressively using musical components

Client independently or interactively invents and performs tonal and/or rhythmic material utilizing overt musical components such as mode, timbre, tempo, phrasing, or dynamic which are congruent with the lyrical content or emotional concept of the improvised music.

xv. Improvises in recognizable musical style
Client independently or interactively invents and performs tonal and/or rhythmic material for one minute or more within a recognizable musical genre, such as blues, gospel, Spanish.

xvi. Improvises in recognizable musical mode
Client independently or interactively invents and performs tonal material for one minute or more within a recognizable musical mode, such as major, minor, pentatonic, Phrygian, or Dorian.

xvii. Creates self-expressive improvisation
Client independently or interactively invents and performs tonal and/or rhythmic material that communicates own feelings, thoughts, or emotions.

H. Music reading

i. Plays simple accompaniment using chord chart
Client plays correct chords on any harmonic instrument from standard written chord chart consisting of two or more chords and at least two measures. No pulse or rhythm required. Simple chord chart is defined as written letters A–G without sharps or flats.

ii. Reads and plays simple rhythmic notation
Client correctly performs rhythms from quarter to whole notes, including rests, using IMTAP Music Sample Hii.

iii. Plays melody of song from written cues
Client plays correct melody of song consisting of at least four differing notes and a minimum of four measures from note names, numbers, or standard music notation. May use IMTAP Music Sample Hiii.

iv. Reads treble clef notation
Client correctly states names of or performs notes from middle C to F within the treble clef staff, not including upper ledger lines, using IMTAP Music Sample Hiv/Hv.

v. Reads and plays music in treble clef notation
Client correctly performs notes from middle C to F within the treble clef staff, not including upper ledger lines, using IMTAP Music Sample Hiv/Hv.

vi. Reads bass clef notation

Client correctly states names of notes or performs notes from G to middle C within the bass clef staff, not including lower ledger lines, using IMTAP Music Sample Hvi/Hvii.

vii. Reads and plays music in bass clef notation

Client correctly performs notes from G to middle C within the bass clef staff, not including lower ledger lines, using IMTAP Music Sample Hvi/Hvii.

viii. Simultaneously reads and plays melody and chords

Client vocally or instrumentally performs a melody and chordal accompaniment from written music consisting of a notated melody line and chord symbols of an entire song structure consisting of at least one verse. An example is singing and playing guitar from written music.

ix. Reads and plays bass and treble clef together

Client correctly performs notes from within the grand staff using IMTAP Music Sample Hix.

I. Accompaniment

i. Accompanies therapist singing/playing

Client provides a musical support on a pitched or un-pitched instrument which is congruent to the therapist's singing or playing, with or without written cues.

ii. Vocalizes and plays simultaneously with pulse

Client sings and performs on pitched or un-pitched instrument with a consistent emphasis on the beats of the music, with or without written cues.

iii. Accompanies self with harmonic instrument

Client plays melody and accompaniment on piano or accompanies own singing using chordal instrument such as guitar, autoharp, piano, or dulcimer, with or without written cues.

Chapter 7

Case Studies

Case Study 1: Neil

Background

Eight-year-old Neil was referred to the music therapy clinic by his parents who requested a specific assessment of their son's musicality. The parents felt it necessary to explore different aspects of their son's potential and musical preferences in consultation with a music therapist before selecting musical instruction or appropriate musical activities. From the music therapy assessment they requested recommendations concerning:

- how to foster Neil's musicality
- ways to enable Neil to develop his skills with success and confidence
- the type of musical instruction or intervention needed
- the role that music might play in Neil's life.

The therapist discussed with the parents the opportunity to assess their son using the newly designed IMTAP process which would provide both specific data and the information they requested.

Intake

Using the IMTAP intake form the therapist recorded information regarding the client in an interview with the referring individual, Neil's mother. Neil had a diagnosis of Asperger syndrome and attention deficit hyperactivity disorder (ADHD). He was not currently taking any medications.

Questions pertaining to the domains of gross motor, fine motor and sensory functioning were all completed with no indications to assess these areas. Although Neil had previously received speech and language therapy services, there were no current indications to assess the receptive or expressive language domains. In the cognitive domain, the IMTAP intake form documented that he was attending mainstream school and was able to work at grade level but occasionally had challenges in remaining focused when completing academic work. In response to questions regarding Neil's social development, his mother reported that he played with typical children and siblings but was more comfortable interacting with younger playmates. Given the indication that there may be concerns in this area, the therapist documented the need to assess the social domain of the IMTAP in addition to the requested musicality domain.

Assessment planning

Neil was seen for three individual sessions at weekly intervals with the same music therapist, and each session was recorded on video for analysis. Sessions contained both pre-planned structured activities and rhythmic or melodic improvisations utilizing a wide range of musical instruments.

Using the IMTAP session outline form, the therapist prepared activities which would directly assess Neil's fundamental skills in the indicated social and musicality domains.

Session I
Activities

1. Greeting song to assess the social fundamentals sub-domain.

2. Exploratory improvisation to assess musicality fundamentals and social skills such as parallel play, imitation, participation, and flexibility.

3. Piano pentatonic improvisation to assess initiation, turn-taking, and call and response.

4. Piano diatonic improvisation over triple-meter ostinato to assess melodic initiation and development.

5. "Let's Find…" blues song finding C, F, and G on the piano to assess participation, attention, and direction following.

6. Pachelbel's *Canon* to assess music reading, direction following, attention, and relationship skills.

7. Electronic synthesizer improvisation to assess exploration of unfamiliar instruments, joint attention, and development of musical ideas.

8. "Goodbye Blues" to assess social fundamentals sub-domain.

In the first session Neil became easily engaged in varying forms of musical interaction including a drum/cymbal improvisation and structured activities at the piano. The therapist introduced a variety of unfamiliar instruments including tone bells, metallophone, and electronic equipment. Neil remained focused and musically interactive for 30 minutes, concluding the first session with simultaneous singing and playing at the drum and cymbal. The session was analyzed and scored as follows.

Musicality domain (MUS)

A. Fundamentals

Once inside the music room Neil was immediately curious about the musical instruments (MUS, Aiii) and spontaneously explored the standing drum and cymbal (MUS, Aiv and Av). As the therapist improvised at the piano to acknowledge and support his steady beating, Neil was consistently alerted by the music (MUS, Ai) and responded by moving rhythmically as he played the drum (MUS, Avii). He consistently expressed his enthusiasm with smiles, gestures, and verbalizations (MUS, Aii).

At the piano, Neil demonstrated consistent engagement in interactive musical play (MUS, Axi) through melodic call and response and spontaneous pentatonic improvisation (MUS, Aviii). Using the tone bells and metallophone, Neil again demonstrated consistent ability to explore unfamiliar instruments (MUS, Av) and play instruments when presented by the therapist (MUS, Aiv). When an electronic synthesizer was introduced, he explored different timbres and ways of playing (MUS, Av) but showed inconsistent interest and desire to play (MUS, Aiii), tending to move quickly through the choices of sounds. This response was noted in the fundamentals sub-domain notes as a personal preference and indicated the future possibility of assessing the IMTAP sensory domain. Neil returned to spontaneous music making at the drum and cymbal (MUS, Aviii), expressing enjoyment by declaring "That was cool" as the session ended (MUS, Aii).

B. Tempo

Within the initial six-minute improvisation at the drum and cymbal, Neil consistently sustained a medium tempo, beating quarter notes in a duple meter (MUS, Bv). When the therapist tested his tolerance and awareness of gross tempo changes (MUS, Bi and Bii) by deliberately contrasting the speed of her piano accompaniment, Neil followed easily and adapted his playing to match the therapist's change of tempo (MUS, Bviii). The therapist then developed the improvisation using differing rhythmic patterns, syncopation, and varied harmonic sequences while Neil began stomping rhythmically and consistently moved his whole body in the tempo of the music (MUS, Biv).

C. Rhythm

In the first session Neil demonstrated consistent rhythmic awareness, imitated simple and intermediate rhythmic patterns of one measure in length (MUS, Ci and Cii), and sustained the imitation of varying rhythmic patterns (MUS, Civ) during turn-taking activities on different instruments with the therapist.

D. Dynamics

Neil consistently demonstrated his awareness of gross dynamic changes by observable differences in the tone of his instrumental playing, changes in affect, and through visual referencing when engaged in improvisation with the therapist (MUS, Di). At the drum, cymbal, and piano he consistently demonstrated a variety of dynamics in his own playing (MUS, Diii) while also tolerating the therapist's use of different dynamics (MUS, Dii). When playing the Pachelbel *Canon* structure using the tone bells and metallophone, he inconsistently followed the therapist's visual cues to alter his dynamic level (MUS, Dv).

E. Vocal

During the final "Goodbye Blues" in F major, Neil began to vocalize in the tonality of the music (MUS, Eiii), completed phrase endings when the therapist paused (MUS, Eiv), and consistently sang the correct melodic pitches of his initiated song (MUS, Evi).

F. Perfect and relative pitch

During the initial assessment session there was no observable indication that Neil possessed relative or perfect pitch. He did not display awareness when the therapist deliberately changed the key of familiar songs, and he did not recognize, match, or name specific pitched tones. In this sub-domain he scored Never for musicality skills Fi, Fiii, Fiv, Fv, Fvi, and Fvii; and scored Inconsistent for his attempts to play in the same tonality as the therapist at the piano (MUS, Fii).

G. Creativity and development of musical ideas

Addressing creative skills was an illuminating part of the IMTAP process for this client. Neil was particularly eager to attempt all the creative activities, showed flexibility in his development of musical ideas and motifs, and was able to be spontaneously creative in the moment.

At the piano, Neil was consistent in his ability to create a melody independently in the pentatonic mode (MUS, Gi), exploring both intervals and step-wise motifs in the treble range. After hearing a four-bar diatonic ostinato he created his own piano melody (MUS, Gix) and was able to develop it independently into an eight-bar structure. In both the pentatonic and diatonic scales, Neil initiated a melodic call and response with the therapist (MUS, Gviii) and improvised within the pentatonic and diatonic modes (MUS, Gxvi). The therapist also made note of his immediate involvement, focused attention, and enthusiasm during the creative opportunities provided in the session.

Social domain (SOC)

On meeting the therapist for the first time, Neil was polite and cooperative. He quickly showed willingness to participate in both structured and unstructured activities, sustaining consistent levels of attention and interaction throughout the session. Neil's social assessment was scored as follows.

A. Fundamentals

Neil responded verbally to his name (SOC, Ai) and demonstrated awareness of the therapist (SOC, Aii) by positioning himself so he had direct eye contact (SOC, Aviii) and could reference the therapist while playing (SOC, Aix). He demonstrated immediate and consistent interest in the presented activities (SOC, Aiii) and used socially appropriate greeting and goodbyes (SOC, Avi and Avii).

B. Participation

Within the initial session Neil displayed consistent levels of participation, entering and remaining in the music situation with ease (SOC, Bi and Bii). He tolerated activity transitions willingly (SOC, Bv) and consistently attempted new tasks, including unfamiliar musical improvisation (SOC, Biii).

C. Turn-taking

Neil sustained rhythmic and melodic turn-taking at both the drum and piano and scored consistently on all items in this sub-domain.

D. Attention

With the exception of the exploration of an electronic instrument, Neil displayed sustained activity-length attention without distraction during the initial session (SOC, Dii and Diii). He maintained consistent attention during a structured bell activity, a note-finding song, and a six-minute rhythmic improvisation (SOC, Di). Throughout the session he consistently demonstrated sustained attention to the therapist (SOC, Diii).

E. Direction following

Neil did not show any difficulties in this sub-domain. He consistently followed one- and two-step verbal directions (SOC, Ei and Eii) concerning the preparation of activities and responded immediately to musical cues (SOC, Eiii).

F. Relationship skills

Neil displayed strong and consistent relationship skills. He easily tolerated direct interaction (SOC, Fi) including conversation and instruction. He appeared comfortable with direct musical contact (SOC, Fiii) such as turn-taking and collaborative improvisation, played in parallel (SOC, Fiv), and consistently imitated musical ideas during piano improvisation (SOC, Fv).

Session 1 summary

The therapist documented her immediate impressions of the initial IMTAP session before reviewing and scoring the assessment using the video tape and IMTAP scoring chart for the musicality and social domains.

In the musicality domain, Neil indicated many areas of consistency including fundamental skills, strong instrumental playing in tempo, imitation of simple and intermediate rhythmic patterns, awareness of dynamic and tempo changes, pitched singing, rhythmic initiation, and melodic initiation.

In assessing the social domain the therapist noted Neil's ease of engagement, consistent levels of sustained participation in both structured activities and improvisation, as well as his tolerance of changes within direct, flexible musical interaction. In contrast to the original intake information, the therapist noted higher levels of social functioning and attention than anticipated.

In preparing for the second assessment session, the therapist deliberately focused on different skills within the social and musicality domains of the IMTAP while also continuing to challenge the skills Neil had demonstrated.

Session 2

Activities

1. Drum/cymbal improvisation to assess responsiveness to changing musical components and flexibility.

2. Autoharp with chord chart to assess music reading, following visual cues and accompaniment skills.

3. Piano note reading to assess music reading.

4. Lyric writing and completing song phrases to assess creativity, flexibility, and cooperation.

5. Vocal improvisation over harmonic support to assess melodic and expressive creativity.

Musicality domain (MUS)

A. Fundamentals

Skills within this sub-domain remained consistent during the second session.

B. Tempo

At the standing drum and cymbal, Neil confidently initiated drumming in his own tempo (MUS, Bv) before initiating tempo changes (MUS, Bvii) in a playful exchange with the therapist and incorporated multiples of the basic beat consistently in his playing (MUS, Bxii). The therapist assessed Neil's responsiveness to changing musical components by changing the piano accompaniment. In this regard, Neil was inconsistent in attempts to follow a gradual accelerando (MUS, Bix) but adjusted to the faster tempo with encouragement. He then maintained consistent playing in the therapist's tempo (MUS, Bvi).

C. Rhythm

During an improvisation using a strong harmonic minor mode, Neil consistently initiated different rhythmic patterns during turn-taking (MUS, Cvii), initiated varying rhythmic structures involving multiple patterns (MUS, Cviii), and sustained self-initiated patterns purposefully (MUS, Cx).

D. Dynamics

During this session, Neil displayed both self-initiated and responsive instrumental playing with a consistent range of dynamic variation (MUS, Diii and Div).

E. Vocal

Neil vocalized enthusiastically in response to a Reggae song style (MUS, Eii) and began to consistently create and develop his own song structure (MUS, Exii) by altering the lyrics, initiating a playful vocal riff and adding an original verse.

G. Creativity and development of musical ideas

Within a lyric writing structure Neil was able to consistently create melodic phrases with harmonic support (MUS, Gix), improvise words to the given rhythmic patterns (MUS, Gvi), and extend the known structure through vocal improvisation (MUS, Gxi).

H. Music reading

In this session the therapist assessed Neil's music reading skills using a written chord chart. Following and selecting the three correct autoharp chords of a familiar song was well within Neil's capabilities and he was consistent in playing the simple accompaniment using a chord chart (MUS, Hi).

At the piano, Neil carefully and consistently played a melody containing six different tones, reading from music notation with letter names identified on the music and keyboard (MUS, Hiii). He was inconsistent when reading and playing the rhythm of the same piece consisting of quarter and half notes (MUS, Hii) and was not able to read treble clef notation when the letter names were omitted (MUS, Hiv). Higher levels of music reading in this sub-domain were recorded as beyond Neil's abilities and were scored as Never (MUS, Hv, Hvi, Hvii, Hviii, and Hix).

I. Accompaniment

Neil consistently accompanied the therapist's singing of a familiar melody by reading a three-chord chart and strumming the autoharp in tempo (MUS, Ii). He tried repeatedly but was inconsistent in attempts to accompany his own singing at the piano and autoharp (MUS, Iii and Iiii).

Social domain (SOC)

A. Fundamentals

In the second session the therapist continued to assess fundamentals of the social domain. During the initial improvisation and the new structured activities, the therapist recorded Neil's consistent joint attention (SOC, Aiv) and appropriate interaction with the therapist (SOC, Av). The therapist noted his consistent display of confidence (SOC, Axii) observed through his body language and his instrumental and vocal responses.

B. Participation

Neil participated consistently in the three new structured activities (SOC, Bvi), showed flexibility in developing the song writing activity and rhythmic improvisation (SOC, Bvii), and demonstrated his ability to work towards identified goals during the session (SOC, Bix).

C. Turn-taking; D. Attention; E. Direction following

Skills within these sub-domains remained at a consistent level during the second session.

F. Relationship skills

Neil came to the second session confidently and sustained two-way communication with the therapist, discussing summer school work and initiating conversation regarding his computer and the musical instruments (SOC, Fvii). During the session he worked cooperatively and consistently with the therapist while demonstrating flexibility within interactive musical play such as improvisation and turn-taking (SOC, Fix).

Session 2 summary

In scoring the second session the therapist noted additional consistent responses in the rhythmic, vocal, and creativity sub-domains. Neil's inconsistent ability to control acceleration in his instrumental playing and his ability to read musical notation with letter names was recorded.

In the social domain the therapist recorded consistent interaction, participation, and flexibility in developing activities. Changes in the initial scoring included increasing Neil's scores in the participation and attention sub-domains.

Session 3

In the final IMTAP session the therapist introduced ostinato/harmonic playing, synchronization of rhythmic patterns, improvisation using different musical motifs to represent pictorial images and extension of Neil's choice of musical instruments to assess further skills in the musicality domain. Within the social domain, the therapist assessed Neil's initiation and ability to extend activities, his ability to take on the leadership role and to move between independent or interdependent skills.

Activities

1. Instrumental improvisation to assess extended use of instruments and development of musical ideas.

2. Introduction of guitar and two chords to assess musicality and accompaniment skills.

3. Ostinato/harmonic playing using three bass tone bars and piano to assess ability to create diatonic melody and bass patterns, flexibility, leadership, and changing roles.

4. Drum and cymbal to assess coordination of two rhythmic patterns.

5. Improvisation to assess independent assignment of differing instruments or musical motifs to express images shown in prepared pictures, creative development, and independent/interdependent skills.

6. "Blues Goodbye".

Musicality domain (MUS)

C. Rhythm

Neil entered the final session and began by initiating a rhythmic structure consisting of drum, cymbal, wind chimes, and tone blocks (MUS, Cviii). He continued to build on his initial musical ideas, consistently using each instrument with clear rhythmic differentiation while developing repeated multiple patterns (MUS, Cix). As the therapist joined his improvisation with a chord progression at the piano, Neil independently began to change rhythmic patterns in response to the music (MUS, Cv) using syncopated and triplet patterns.

As Neil was confident in his use of multiple musical instruments the therapist introduced an activity synchronizing two rhythmic patterns simultaneously (MUS, Cvi). To the therapist's surprise, this was the first indication of a real challenge within the rhythm sub-domain. In triple time Neil was not able to sustain his playing, and in duple time he repeatedly worked at coordinating the two given patterns. He accomplished it finally after sustained attempts, prompts, and additional musical support but received a score of Rarely for this skill, displaying less than 50 percent attainment.

D. Dynamics

During the initial improvisation Neil demonstrated the ability to consistently adapt his playing to control crescendos in response to the piano's rising chromaticism (MUS, Dvi). As Neil and the therapist changed roles with each other creating a diatonic piano melody over ostinato patterns played on the bass tone bars, Neil continued to display awareness of dynamics in his playing (MUS, Di), consistently decreasing the volume of his playing in response to the therapist's quieter dynamics (MUS, Dvii).

E. Vocal

In the final session Neil spontaneously vocalized in the same tonality as the initial instrumental improvisation (MUS, Ev) and again extended the "Goodbye" song. He began to create and consistently develop his own song structure (MUS, Exii), singing "Music today, it'll always be here, in your heart." During this self-expressive lyrical improvisation (MUS, Exi) the therapist recorded Neil's consistent singing which displayed his sensitivity to musical components including changing tempo, phrasing, and dynamics (MUS, Evii).

G. Creativity and development of musical ideas

For the final IMTAP activity the therapist introduced a choice of three photos for Neil to express using a wide range of percussive and tuned instruments. First Neil chose a picture of penguins in the snow and independently assigned the wind chimes and high pentatonic piano clusters to depict the cold, then a three-note xylophone pattern to represent walking. Wanting to choose another theme, he created a thunderstorm using the piano "with the dark keys" creating clusters which gradually moved higher up the keyboard and then bursts of loud drumming as the storm retreated. The therapist recorded Neil's enthusiastic ability to consistently assign both differentiated instruments (MUS, Giii) and differentiated musical motifs to given images (MUS, Giv). Although Neil was able to identify his use of musical components to illustrate the images, he was not able to transcribe his ideas using symbols or notation, therefore scoring Never for this skill (MUS, Gxiii).

Social domain (SOC)

A. Fundamentals

During the final session Neil continued to maintain his consistent scoring in the fundamentals sub-domain. Neil demonstrated his consistent awareness of appropriate physical space (SOC, Axi) by adjusting his proximity to the therapist at the piano bench, when sharing musical instruments and when moving from one activity to another. Neil demonstrated consistent confidence (SOC, Axii) throughout the IMTAP process, ending the final session by singing "Music's in your heart, forever," adding "Yes, I had a great time," before leaving the music room.

B. Participation

Neil continued to display consistent and enthusiastic levels of participation during his final assessment session. He consistently initiated new activities when given the opportunity (SOC, Biv), such as independently beginning the initial improvisation and then creating an original vocal structure. His consistent ability to extend all activities appropriately with full participation was recorded by the therapist (SOC, Bviii).

F. Relationship skills

During the final session the therapist assessed Neil's ability to change roles with the therapist. During an activity where the therapist and Neil alternated between providing an ostinato on the bass tone bars or a melody at the piano, Neil consistently worked cooperatively with the therapist (SOC, Fviii) and demonstrated flexibility within the interactive structure (SOC, Fix) by changing musical roles. While depicting visual images using musical instruments, Neil consistently assumed the leadership role (SOC, Fxi) by organizing the materials, discussing his ideas, and directing the therapist to listen and observe.

Session 3 summary

In the final session Neil continued to display consistent scores across multiple sub-domains of the social and musicality domains. In the third session his only challenge appeared when attempting to synchronize two different rhythmic patterns simultaneously. In the social domain Neil rose to the challenges of leadership and appeared consistently comfortable and flexible in his musical interactions with the therapist.

IMTAP summary (Neil)

Before reviewing the IMTAP results with Neil's parents the therapist completed all scoring of the musicality and social domains (Figure 7.1) and documented his strengths and needs using the IMTAP summary sheet.

The IMTAP process was clearly a positive and motivating experience for Neil. His mother commented that she had observed his ability to be creative, to clearly develop his ideas, and to attend to unfamiliar activities. She acknowledged that the combination of structured activities and improvisational material had enabled her to observe newly identified skill levels with multiple examples of his musical responsiveness and potential. Socially, she was surprised at how comfortable Neil appeared in each session, and that he was able to approach each activity, challenge, or experience willingly. She remarked on the unique opportunity for Neil to focus and channel his energy using movement, vocalizations and instrumental responses within shared musical interaction. Overall, she was surprised that her son had been able to display spontaneity and confidence in an unfamiliar assessment situation. Viewing the IMTAP scores and graph confirmed her observations and clarified her consideration of his individual potential.

After three individual 30-minute sessions the therapist was confident that the IMTAP had provided multiple opportunities to assess Neil's musical and social skills and had highlighted areas for potential development. In this situation the therapist found the implementation of the IMTAP particularly useful in ensuring that a comprehensive range of skill levels were addressed within a variety of musical activities and experiences. The identified skills documented in the IMTAP enabled the therapist to systematically build on Neil's fundamental abilities and innate responses while offering specific challenges in each sub-domain. Neil's final domain and sub-domain graphs (Figures 7.1, 7.2, and 7.3) displayed strong musical and social skills across all domains with identified needs that could be addressed further using the modality of music.

The IMTAP was used to provide information for the family to use in selecting musical instruction. In review with the family, the therapist first acknowledged the parents in following their instincts and seeking a comprehensive music therapy assessment for their son. The music therapist made the following recommendations:

1. Involvement in a children's choir, which included singing, music reading, performing, and an opportunity for participation in a new social situation.

2. Referral to a local music therapist/teacher who would provide piano lessons, music reading, improvisation, rhythmic activities, and duet work.

3. Participation in a children's drum circle with peers and siblings.

4. Exploration of musical software, utilizing technology to create, record and notate original compositions.

5. Exposure to a wide variety of musical experiences and differing musical styles.

6. Future assessment of sensory responses in reference to electronic musical instruments as well as joint consultation with a sensory integration specialist.

7. Future exploration of guitar lessons.

IMTAP Music Therapy

Neil   D.O.B. 1/21/1998
        Assessment date(s): 7/4/06, 7/11/06, 7/18/06

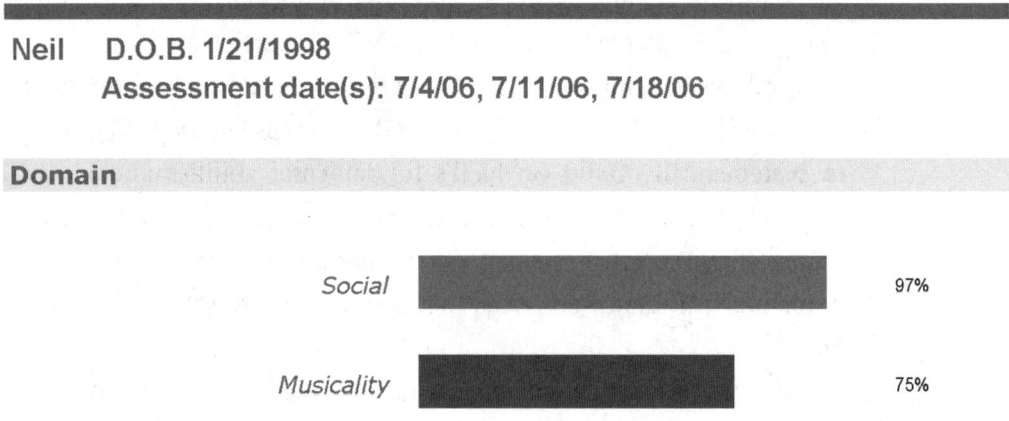

Figure 7.1 Neil's sub-domain profile

IMTAP Music Therapy

Neil   D.O.B. 1/21/1998
        Assessment date(s): 7/4/06, 7/11/06, 7/18/06

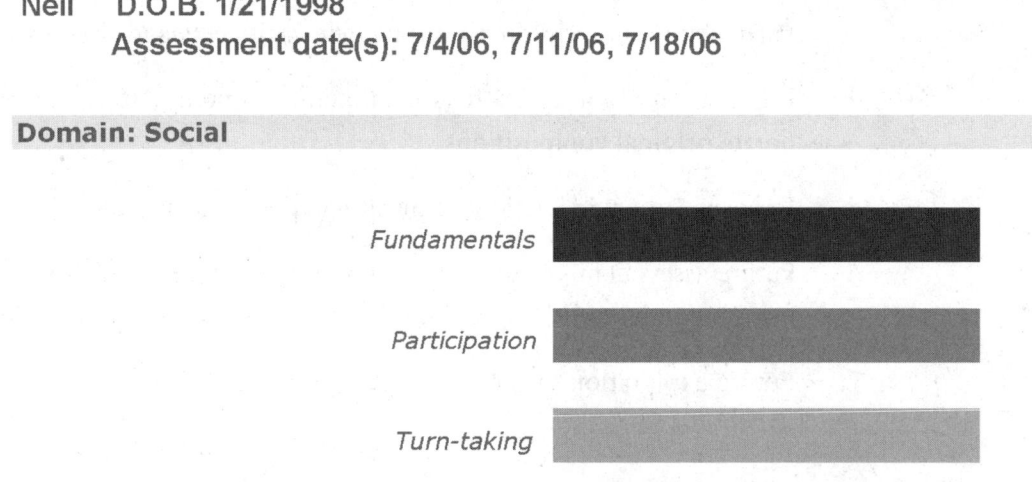

Figure 7.2 Neil's sub-domain profile for social skills

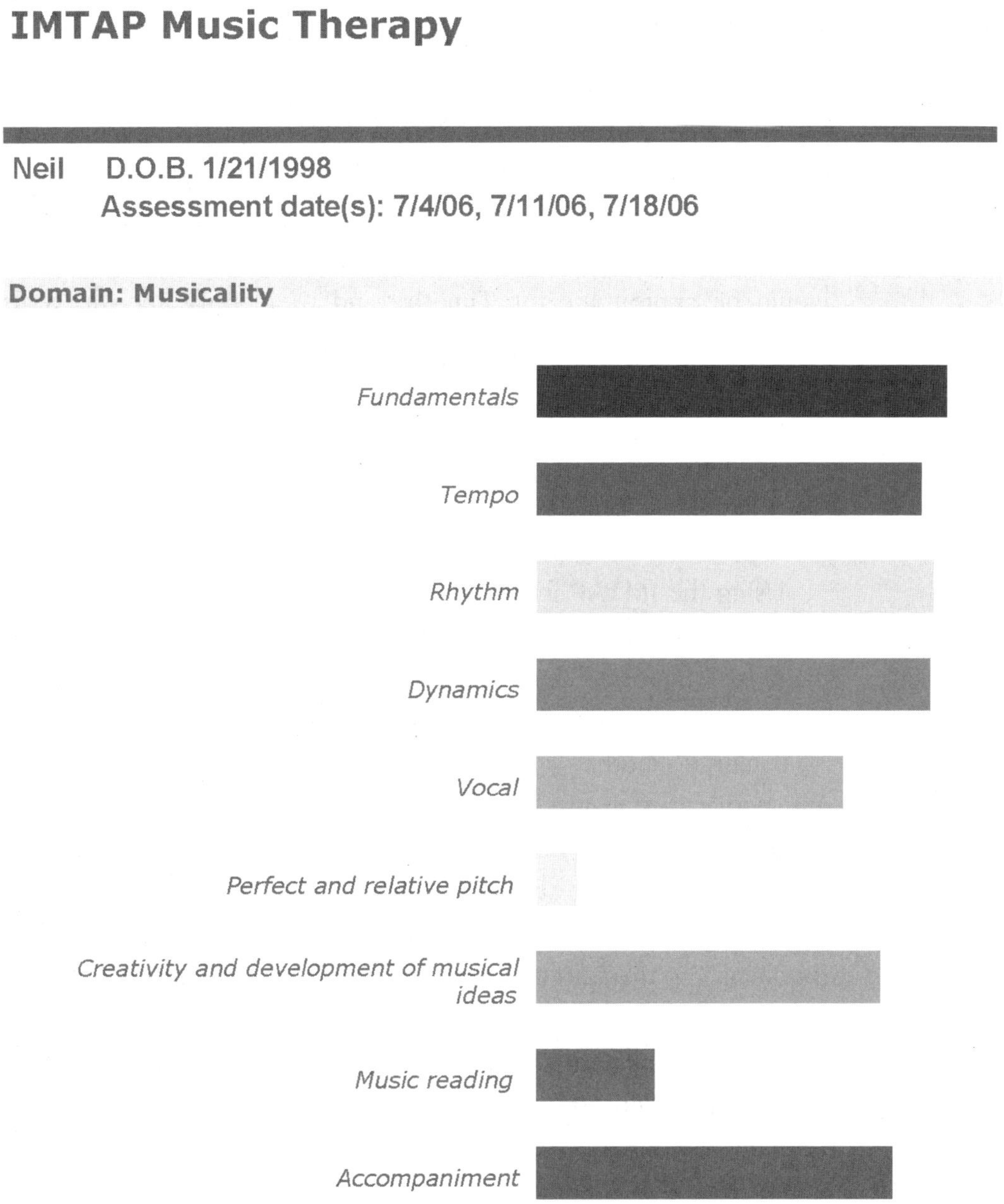

IMTAP Music Therapy

Neil   D.O.B. 1/21/1998
        Assessment date(s): 7/4/06, 7/11/06, 7/18/06

Domain: Musicality

Figure 7.3 Neil's sub-domain profile for musicality

Case Study 2: Timothy

Background

Twelve-year-old Timothy was referred to the music therapy clinic by his parents who requested music therapy services in order to encourage him to try new activities, to develop his awareness of others in social situations, and to decrease his sensitivities to sounds. The IMTAP was administered to determine whether music therapy services would be appropriate for Timothy and to identify specific goals that could be addressed.

Intake

Considering the breadth of domains which were assessed, description of the intake scoring has been synopsized by sub-domain.

Using the IMTAP intake form, the therapist recorded information regarding the client in an interview with the referring individual, Timothy's mother. Timothy had a diagnosis of autism. Timothy's mother reported that Timothy was high functioning and was taking two medications for behavior and attention.

Timothy's mother gave complete answers when asked the questions on the intake, which gave the therapist ample information for planning the initial assessment sessions. It was reported that it was important for Timothy to understand what was expected of him and to know the specific activities he would be doing during each session. In addition, Timothy's mother reported that Timothy had intense interests in animals and the circus. The therapist used this information to create activities that would support the development of a strong rapport with the therapist.

The domains of gross motor and oral motor skills were completed on the intake with no indications to assess these areas. In the fine motor domain, it was reported that Timothy had difficulty with writing and tying his shoe laces, but was able to complete those tasks.

In the sensory domain, Timothy's mother reported that he had difficulty tolerating different textures on clothing and that he engaged in repetitive behaviors such as hand flapping when anxious or excited. She also reported that Timothy made "funny noises" and repeated phrases from movies. According to his mother, Timothy had sensitivities to sounds and often placed his hands over his ears when confronted with loud sounds.

In the receptive communication/auditory processing domain, there were no indications that this area needed to be assessed, but Timothy's mother elaborated on the questions stating that Timothy had comprehension and cognitive difficulties. Given this information, the therapist decided to assess this area.

The expressive communication domain indicated several areas of concern. Specifically, Timothy's mother reported that he had a small vocabulary, others had difficulty understanding him, and, although he was capable of communicating effectively, he demonstrated idiosyncratic speech consisting of repetitive phrases.

Timothy's mother reported that Timothy had an Individualized Education Plan (IEP) and demonstrated cognitive deficits. Timothy attended a special education school for children with high functioning autism and Asperger's syndrome.

The emotional and social domains also had several indications that these areas needed to be assessed further. Timothy's mother gave complete answers, elaborating on the questions asked. She reported that he had emotional difficulties and angered easily, especially when interacting with his father and when dealing with feeding issues. She reported that he did not like it when others were upset with him. Socially, Timothy's mother reported that he had many difficulties. She stated that Timothy preferred the company of adults and girls, but did not get along well with boys his age. He did not initiate play with others and participated in conversations only if it was a topic of interest to him.

Given the information gathered during the intake process, it was determined that the domains of fine motor, sensory, receptive communication/auditory processing, cognitive, emotional, social, and musicality would be assessed.

Assessment planning

Timothy was seen for three 30-minute sessions, one time per week by the same music therapist. Each session was recorded on video for analysis. Sessions contained both pre-planned activities and opportunities for improvisation, utilizing a wide range of musical instruments and styles.

Using the IMTAP session outline form the therapist prepared activities which would directly assess Timothy's skills in the selected domains.

Session 1 activities

1. Greeting song to assess social fundamentals, fine motor fundamentals, sensory fundamentals, expressive and receptive communication, auditory perception, and musicality.

2. Animal book sung to assess attention span and areas of musicality such as following simple musical cues and repeating simple rhythmic patterns.

3. Drum improvisation with piano accompaniment to assess awareness of gross changes in tempo, dynamic, and meter as well as participation, direction following, awareness of sound versus silence, and ability to play in tempo with therapist and imitate simple and intermediate rhythmic patterns.

4. "We're on Our Way to Hear the Band" to assess ability to recall new information, understand rules and structures, as well as the tactile sub-domain of sensory skills.

5. Xylophone improvisation to assess social skills such as playing in parallel with the therapist, playing in imitation of the therapist and sustaining musical interaction, as well as the pitched percussion sub-domain of fine motor skills.

6. Goodbye song to assess participation and willingness to expand on structures.

Session 2 activities

1. Co-development of written activity plan for the session to assess decision making skills, flexibility, interest in repeating activities from the previous session, and willingness to attempt new tasks when given the opportunity.

2. Greeting song to assess long-term recall as well as ability to recall the therapist's name.

3. Song writing based on pictures of Timothy's favorite television shows to assess ability to sustain two-way conversation, creativity, and development of ideas.

4. Guitar strumming to familiar song structure to assess strumming and ability to play in tempo.

5. Drumming imitation to assess musical interaction and ability to imitate simple and intermediate rhythms and follow musical cues.

6. High-five song to assess ability to sequence several steps and the vestibular and proprioceptive sub-domains of the sensory domain.

7. Pentatonic piano improvisation to assess ability to play without splaying, ability to coordinate both hands, and ability to play melodically in tonality of an improvisation.

8. Goodbye song to assess quality of vocalizations and ability to match pitch.

Session 3 activities

1. Note writing with labeled piano keys to assess note reading, choice making, and ability to develop musical ideas.

2. Musical story to assess decision making, creativity, and abstract thinking.

3. Instrumental improvisation to assess ability to explore external social relationships, emotional expression, recognition of emotional states, and ability to communicate emotional content ideas and concepts.

4. Paddle drum to assess playing instruments when presented, turn-taking, and ability to take the leadership role in an activity.

5. Electronic guitar with lighted buttons to assess fine motor skills, attention, and flexibility.

6. Goodbye song on drums and guitar to assess vocal quality and long-term recall.

Fine motor domain (FM)

A. Fundamentals

Timothy scored a Consistent rating on all areas of this sub-domain other than organizing alternate hands in playing (FM, Axi), on which he scored Inconsistent due to his difficulty in sustaining playing in tempo on the pentatonic xylophone and drums.

B. Strumming

The strumming sub-domain was assessed using the guitar and autoharp. Timothy strummed consistently with his whole hand (FM, Bi), but never strummed with a pulse (FM, Biii, Biv, and Bvi). He inconsistently strummed the guitar with his thumb (FM, Bii), as he continued to resort to strumming with his whole hand. Timothy inconsistently strummed with a pick (FM, Bv) as he did not use a pick with the guitar, but did use a pick while strumming the autoharp.

C. Autoharp/Q Chord

Timothy chose to play the autoharp when he created his activity plan for the session, but when the therapist presented it to him, Timothy told the therapist he did not want to play it. The therapist encouraged him to try it, which he did, but had difficulty selecting and pressing a single button (FM, Cii) and never coordinated press and strum (FM, Ciii), so therefore he never followed a chord chart (FM, Civ). Timothy scored Inconsistent on "explores chord buttons" (FM, Ci) as he rarely depressed a single button on cue, but ran his fingers across the buttons and explored the body of the autoharp.

D. Guitar/dulcimer

Timothy demonstrated interest in the guitar from the first session as evidenced by his asking what it was and if he could play it. Timothy held the guitar and strummed it with an open hand and was able to strum while holding a pick. Timothy never strummed with a pulse and scored Never on "approximates simple chords" (FM, Dii) as assessed by using a guitar with buttons that light up to indicate simple chord positions. Timothy did not play individual strings (FM, Dvi) when the therapist asked him to imitate the therapist's plucking of single strings.

E. Piano

Timothy's highest scores in this sub-domain were Inconsistent ratings on "uses fingers of dominant hand without splaying" (FM, Cii) and "uses single finger of dominant hand" (FM, Civ). This was assessed using a piano improvisation with instructions for Timothy to play the black keys as well as asking Timothy to imitate the therapist's playing. Timothy never sequenced fingers (FM, Evi and Evii), formed triads (FM, Eviii and Eix), or coordinated his hands (FM, Ei).

F. Pitched percussive/mallet

Timothy played the pentatonic marimba with the therapist and did not demonstrate an awareness of different pitched tones, which the therapist then scored as Never on "plays isolated note with mallet" (FM, Fii). Instead, he played it as if it were a drum. Timothy never sequenced a pattern of notes (FM, Fiv), or rhythmic pattern (FM, Fiv). Timothy did match the number of beats in imitation and this was noted by the therapist.

Receptive communication/auditory perception domain (RC)

A. Fundamentals

Timothy scored Consistent on the lower level skills in this section as he demonstrated awareness of sound vs. silence (RC, Ai) and localized sound directionality (RC, Aii and Aiii) as evidenced by asking for more when the music stopped and looking toward the guitar when the therapist began playing. However, Timothy scored Never on the higher level skills. During a xylophone improvisation, Timothy never imitated a simple musical motif (RC, Av) initiated by the therapist. Timothy continued to score Consistent for the lower level skills and Rarely/Never on the higher level skills throughout the remainder of the receptive communication sub-domains.

B. Direction following

Timothy followed both one- and two-step directions (RC, Bi and Bii) when presented in a song structure and when presented verbally. When engaged in a drumming activity of playing and stopping, Timothy only stopped and started when the therapist sang the direction; he did not follow an instrumental cue or musical cadence to stop, warranting a score of Rarely on "follows simple musical cues" (RC, Biii).

C. Musical changes

The musical changes sub-domain was assessed using piano/drum improvisations. Timothy seemed to struggle in this area as he did not show an awareness of mutual musical interaction as evidenced by rarely changing his playing to demonstrate an awareness of gross tempo, pitch, or dynamic changes (RC, Ci, Cii, and Ciii). He never demonstrated awareness of meter changes (RC, Civ) and never demonstrated awareness of changes in intensity/mood (RC, Cv). Timothy never played melodically in the key (RC, Cvi). Even when instructed to play "just the black keys," Timothy did not sustain that interaction and moved to both the black and white keys.

D. Singing/vocalizing

During the greeting and goodbye songs, Timothy vocalized along with the music therapist, echoing each phrase, warranting a score of Consistent on "vocalizes in response to aural stimuli" (RC, Di), "vocalizes in response to therapist speaking" (RC, Dii), and "vocalizes in response to therapist singing" (RC, Diii). He also consistently vocalized in provided musical pauses (RC, Dix). Timothy scored Rarely and Never for the remainder of this sub-domain. Timothy sang in key (RC, Dviii) when presented with familiar songs, but did not sing in key along with newly learned songs, warranting a score of Rarely. He did not demonstrate any specific responses to particular idioms, modes, or motifs (RC, Dvi), warranting a score of Never. This was assessed through pentatonic marimba improvisations as well as piano and instrumental improvisations using the Spanish and Middle Eastern idiom.

E. Rhythm

Timothy had several opportunities to play along with the therapist using drums, a xylophone, piano, guitar, and other rhythm instruments. He needed a great deal of support in order to play in tempo (RC, Ei), indicating an Inconsistent score. Timothy neither matched the therapist's rhythms nor established his own internal beat. For example, Timothy played in tempo with the therapist if the therapist strummed quarter notes on the guitar while Timothy played the drum. However, if the therapist played eighth notes or any multiple of quarter notes, Timothy did not sustain the tempo. Timothy imitated simple rhythmic patterns on the drum (RC, Eii) if he counted along with the therapist and counted while he played or if the therapist added a syllable, such as "boom" to the playing, warranting a score of Inconsistent. Timothy never imitated intermediate rhythmic patterns (RC, Eiii).

Expressive communication domain (EC)

A. Fundamentals

When first communicating with Timothy, it appeared that expressive communication would not be an area of difficulty. He consistently communicated clearly upon verbally greeting the therapist and during the greeting song and never demonstrated frustration when communicating (EC, Aii). Upon further examination, however, Timothy rarely communicated ideas and concepts (EC, Aiv) and rarely communicated emotional content and idea development (EC, Av). This was demonstrated during several activities including an instrumental improvisation during which Timothy was asked to assign an instrument to an emotion and play the chosen instrument to express that emotion. Timothy answered "I don't know" to all of the questions included in this activity such as, "Which instrument sounds happy/sad/excited/angry, etc.?"

B. Non-vocal communication

This section was marked N/A as Timothy communicates verbally.

C. Vocalizations

Timothy scored Inconsistent on "vocalizations are of clear tonal quality" (EC, Ci) as his speaking voice and his singing voice were, on occasion, nasal sounding. In addition, he scored Inconsistent on "vocalizations are of appropriate volume" (EC, Cii) and "vocalizations are of moderate pitch range" (EC, Ciii) as his voice tended to be loud and "sing-songy."

D. Spontaneous vocalizations

Timothy consistently vocalized with the therapist (EC, Di) during several singing activities, but never vocalized spontaneously during instrumental activities, warranting an Inconsistent score. Upon introducing new songs, Timothy echoed the therapist after each phrase. He sang and read along with the therapist when participating in a sung book activity. When involved in singing, Timothy's vocalizations were nearly always imitative, but purposeful, as evidenced by his engagement in the activity and echoing the song lyrics being presented in the ongoing activity, warranting a score of Consistent on "vocalizations are purposefully imitative" (EC, Diii) and Inconsistent on "vocalizations are of non-imitative type" (EC, Dii).

E. Verbalizations

Timothy scored Consistent on all of the areas in this section as he had no difficulty with intelligibility or creating full length phrases or sentences.

F. Relational communication

Timothy had difficulty in this area as he demonstrated anxiety when involved in direct interaction with the therapist. This was evidenced by hand wringing, shifting his weight back and forth, and by attempting to change the subject. He answered most closed questions (EC, Fi) by saying either "I don't know" or "okay." When asked binary questions (EC, Fii), such as the ones asked when participating in a sung book that involved assigning instruments to different sounds in the book, Timothy had even greater difficulty making the choice, warranting an Inconsistent score. Regarding asking questions, Timothy consistently asked questions (EC, Fv) about the appropriate way to play the instruments, but he rarely asked other questions, warranting an Inconsistent score. Timothy rarely initiated conversation (EC, Fiv).

G. Vocal idiosyncrasies

Timothy did not demonstrate any vocal idiosyncrasies. There were rare occasions when his vocalizations were scripted (EC, Gvi), as he repeated phrases initiated by his mother.

Cognitive domain (COG)

A. Fundamentals

Timothy was inconsistent in his ability to sustain-activity length attention span (COG, Ai). His ability seemed dependent upon his motivation to participate in an activity. For example, during drumming and improvisational play, Timothy sustained his attention, but during activities such as song writing that required Timothy to choose notes on the keyboard, he scored Inconsistent in sustaining his attention. It was noted that even while participating in activities that seemed enjoyable to him, Timothy often asked "What's next?" Timothy demonstrated consistent ability to understand rules and structures (COG, Aiii). This was assessed through the introduction of several games that required listening to directions prior to participation.

B. Decision making

This was an area of great difficulty for Timothy. At the beginning of each session, Timothy was given a list of choices to determine which activities would occur that day (COG, Bii and Biii). He completed his activity plan without difficulty, but during the actual activities he struggled with decision making. This was especially apparent during a song writing activity where Timothy was asked to choose notes from the keyboard and write them on a white board to be read back and played. Timothy became visibly anxious when asked to choose the notes. He wanted to know exactly how many notes he needed to choose and when the activity was going to end. He completed the task with several prompts and with tremendous support from the therapist; therefore, Timothy scored Rarely on "makes choices between three presented concrete options" (COG, Biii) and "makes choices without prompting" (COG, Bv). Timothy previously scored Inconsistent on the cross-domain skill "answers binary questions" (EC, Fii), so this sub-domain was scored accordingly.

C. Direction following

This cross-domain skill was assessed, scored, and described in the receptive communication/auditory processing domain.

D. Short-term recall/sequencing

Timothy consistently recalled new information within the introduced activities (COG, Di). This was assessed through an instrumental activity that required Timothy to remember the names of instruments and play them when indicated in the song. During another activity that required Timothy to remember a sequence of instruments to be played along with a story book, he was inconsistent in his ability to remember the sequence of activities, but with support and prompting he recalled several instruments in consecutive order (COG, Dii and Diii), indicating scores of Inconsistent.

E. Long-term recall

Timothy scored Consistent on the lower-level skills in this sub-domain other than in his ability to recall the therapist's name (COG, Ei), on which he scored Never. He demonstrated an inconsistent awareness of the music therapy routine (COG, Eiv) as Timothy required an activity plan at the start of each session. After the first session, it was clear that Timothy recalled the functions of instruments and their names as evidenced by consistently requesting them by name during subsequent sessions (COG, Eii, and Eiii). Timothy never participated in reading or playing accompaniment (COG, Evii, Eviii, and Eix).

F. Academics

This sub-domain was not assessed as the therapist did not have the time to incorporate all tasks in this area within the first three sessions. It was noticed, however, that Timothy could read, recognize numbers and colors, and write full words.

Sensory domain (SEN)
A. Fundamentals

Timothy consistently integrated sensory information of multiple types (SEN, Ai and Aii) as evidenced by sustained attention and regulation during all musical activities.

B. Tactile

Timothy scored Consistent on all areas of this sub-domain. He participated in several tactile activities including tolerating putting a mouthpiece to his lips (SEN, Bvi), playing a cabasa, and strumming a guitar. He remained physically open to the presentation of all instruments (SEN, Bix) and played each instrument appropriately and without difficulty.

C. Proprioceptive

This area was assessed using a song that required several types of movement. Timothy demonstrated ability to start/stop each movement and remained on-task throughout the song (SEN, Cii, Ciii, and Civ), warranting Consistent scores in this sub-domain.

D. Vestibular

The aforementioned song was used to assess this sub-domain and Timothy showed consistent abilities in all areas.

E. Visual

Timothy scored Consistent in all of the areas of this sub-domain other than "retains gaze of object or person for appropriate length of time" (SEN, Evi). The therapist observed that Timothy sustained inconsistent eye contact with the therapist and others. As Timothy did not demonstrate other difficulties in this area and did not demonstrate this difficulty with gaze of objects, it was concluded that the inconsistent eye contact was related to social difficulties.

F. Auditory

Timothy's scores fell between Consistent and Inconsistent in this area. He scored Inconsistent in the areas of stopping an auditory activity (SEN, Fv) and demonstrating an awareness of sound vs. silence (SEN, Fii). Timothy consistently attended to auditory tasks (SEN, Fvi) and demonstrated abilities to return to task after most auditory distractions without prompts (SEN, Fviii). As he could return to task after auditory distractions without prompts, the previous skill "returns to task after auditory distractions with prompts" (SEN, Fvii) was scored as Consistent.

Social domain (SOC)

A. Fundamentals

Timothy consistently responded to his own name and demonstrated awareness of the therapist (SOC, Ai and Aii). His interest in activities was scored Inconsistent, dependent upon the difficulty of the task. The more difficult the task, the less interest Timothy displayed (SOC, Aiii). He consistently demonstrated joint attention while playing instruments with the therapist, but rarely demonstrated joint attention on the music being played (SOC, Aiv) indicating a score of Inconsistent. Timothy used socially appropriate greetings (SOC, Avi and Avii) but had inconsistent eye contact throughout the sessions (SOC, Aviii). He referenced his mother when she was in the room, saying that he was playing for her (SOC, Aviii) and inconsistently referenced the therapist. Timothy displayed some anxiety and lack of confidence in the music therapy setting (SOC, Axii) when asked to make decisions, expand activities, or stray from his activity plan.

B. Participation

Timothy was cooperative throughout all three assessment sessions as he consistently entered the room and remained in the room for the duration of each session (SOC, Bi and Bii). Timothy attempted new tasks (SOC, Biii) only if they had been written on his session schedule, therefore he scored Inconsistent. On one occasion Timothy requested the guitar even though it was not on his activity plan, indicating a score of Rarely on "initiates new activity when given opportunity" (SOC, Biv). Timothy consistently participated in all structured activities presented (SOC, Bvi), but never allowed for the development of activities (SOC, Bvii). For example, after Timothy became familiar with a sung animal book, the therapist suggested adding movements to the verses. Timothy declined to participate in this expansion of the activity.

C. Turn-taking

Timothy scored consistently on all tasks in this sub-domain. This area was assessed using a structured paddle drum activity.

D. Attention

Timothy inconsistently sustained activity-length attention span (SOC, Di) depending on his interest and comfort level with the activity. As a cross-domain skill, this information was also gathered in the cognitive fundamentals sub-domain. On most occasions, Timothy returned to activities without prompts (SOC, Dii), scoring Consistent on this task, but there were instances when he was involved in more challenging activities requiring prompts for Timothy to stay on task (SOC, Di), warranting a score of Inconsistent.

E. Direction following

As a cross-domain skill, this information was gathered and described in the receptive language/auditory processing domain under sub-domain B.

F. Relationship skills

The majority of activities presented in the assessment sessions were used to evaluate this sub-domain. Timothy's abilities were splintered in this area as he scored Consistent in the first three tasks: tolerates direct interaction (SOC, Fi), redirection (SOC, Fii), and musical contact (SOC, Fiii). Timothy also consistently played in parallel with the therapist (SOC, Fiv), but did not seem to make the connection of mutual music making, so although the therapist was involved with Timothy's playing, he was quite independent in his playing. For this reason, Timothy scored Never on "sustains musical interaction" (SOC, Fvi). While Timothy was consistently cooperative with the therapist (SOC, Fviii), he rarely demonstrated flexibility within familiar interactive structures such as expanding improvisations or instrumental activities (SOC, Fx). Timothy also had great difficulty exploring external social relationships (SOC, Fxiii), indicating a score of Never. This was evident during an instrumental improvisation focusing on emotional exploration. After each improvisation, Timothy was asked several questions about situations and people that elicit emotions. He answered all questions with "I don't know," and then requested to move on to the next task and asked how many more times he had to do the task.

Emotional domain (EMO)

A. Affect

Timothy showed a limited range of affect within each session (EMO, Ai and Aiii), indicating a score of Rarely. It was unclear whether this was due to limited ability in this area or due to Timothy's pleasant mood throughout each session. He was inconsistent in demonstrating appropriate affect (EMO, Aii) in that during activities that were challenging, he continued smiling, but demonstrated other signs of anxiety. In addition, while smiling and expressing his enjoyment in activities, he was also asking when he was going to be able to finish the task.

B. Differentiation/expression

Timothy rarely expressed emotions appropriate to circumstances (EMO, Bi). When asked if he was happy or enjoying himself, Timothy always answered "yes," even when he was asking to stop an activity. He did not express his emotions verbally (EMO, Biii) or with instruments (EMO, Bii), warranting scores of Never. When presented with various improvisations and structured instrumental activities, Timothy did not demonstrate emotional sensitivity to musical components (EMO, Biv), warranting a score of Never.

C. Regulation

Timothy did not demonstrate difficulty in this area as he remained regulated throughout the sessions. It was noted, however, that prior to each session and at the end of each session, Timothy became very physical with his mother by pushing and tickling her. He then used scripted language to say "I don't like that. Control yourself." His scores ranged from Inconsistent to Consistent in all of the areas of this sub-domain.

D. Self-awareness

Timothy showed little to no self-awareness during the assessment sessions. He rarely demonstrated recognition of emotional states (EMO, Di) as evidenced by his difficulty discussing pictures of emotions. He also never demonstrated the ability to explore or discuss emotional states (EMO, Dii and Diii). He demonstrated avoidance when presented with opportunities to discuss emotional content and never initiated interactions around emotional topics (EMO, Div). Due to low scores in these earlier skills, the final skill "demonstrates desire to better oneself or life circumstances" (EMO, Dv) was scored Never without being directly assessed within the session.

Musicality domain (MUS)

A. Fundamentals

Timothy scored in the Consistent range for all areas of this sub-domain other than "moves rhythmically in response to music" (MUS, Avi), "engages in interactive musical play" (MUS, Axi), and "regulates with musical support" (MUS, Axii), on which he scored Never or Rarely. He scored an Inconsistent on the cross-domain skill "responds to musical cues" (MUS, Ax) as he required a sung or verbal cue in addition to the musical cue.

B. Tempo

Timothy tolerated tempo changes (MUS, Bi) as it did not appear to the music therapist that he was aware of the changes. Timothy scored Never or Rarely for the remainder of this sub-domain as he did not adapt his playing (MUS, Bxi, Bxii, Bxiii, and Bxiv), sustain playing (MUS, Bx), or initiate tempo changes (MUS, Bvii).

C. Rhythm

Timothy consistently imitated simple rhythmic patterns (MUS, Ci), but inconsistently imitated intermediate patterns unless accompanied by a vocal cue (MUS, Cii). He scored Never for the remainder of this category as he did not sustain (MUS, Civ), change (MUS, Cv), coordinate (MUS, Cvi), develop (MUS, Cix), or initiate (MUS, Cviii) rhythmic patterns or structures. When involved in rhythmic playing, Timothy either imitated patterns or played a drum roll.

D. Dynamics

Timothy tolerated changing dynamics (MUS, Dii) as it did not appear to the therapist that he was aware of the change. On one occasion when the therapist initiated a softer dynamic, Timothy said "louder" and continued to play loudly. He scored Never on the remaining areas other than "follows cue to change dynamic" (MUS, Dv), on which he scored Inconsistent as he did follow verbal directions from the therapist.

E. Vocal

Timothy consistently vocalized to complete known song phrases (MUS, Eiv), but rarely sang in the key (MUS, Ev) unless the song was extremely familiar to him, such as "Row Row Row Your Boat." He scored Never on the remaining items in this sub-domain.

F. Perfect and relative pitch

Timothy scored Never on all areas of this sub-domain as there was no evidence that he had perfect or relative pitch.

G. Creativity and development of musical ideas

While the therapist attempted to assess this section, Timothy did not demonstrate any abilities to complete these tasks, other than to assign differentiated instruments to given ideas or images (MUS, Giv) as he participated in adding sound effects to a sung story on which he scored Inconsistent. The majority of the skills in this domain were scored as Never.

H. Music reading

Timothy scored Never on all areas of this sub-domain as he did not demonstrate skills needed to introduce this subject.

I. Accompaniment

Although the therapist attempted to assess this sub-domain, Timothy scored Rarely and Never in all three areas.

IMTAP summary (Timothy)

From the intake to the development of goals and objectives, the IMTAP was an excellent resource for gathering thorough information about Timothy. The complete answers given by Timothy's mother during the intake allowed the therapist to determine the appropriate domains to assess. Because of the comprehensive questions on the intake, the therapist was able to gather additional information about Timothy that his mother did not initially identify as being an area of need. Specifically, Timothy's mother reported minor difficulties with receptive communication. With further discussion, the intake process cued the therapist to assess this domain which did, in fact, prove to be of significant value in identifying Timothy's goals in therapy.

The intake process also revealed that the sensory domain was an area to be assessed. Because of the cross-domain skill (retains eye gaze) in the sensory and social domains, the therapist was able to determine that Timothy's difficulty in this area was related to difficulty with social skills rather than to a visual sensory problem. In addition, Timothy's mother reported that he had sound sensitivity. The assessment process indicated that Timothy tolerated a variety of sensory input and was able to consistently integrate sensory information. In addition, changes in sound quality such as dynamic and musical mode appeared to have no effect on Timothy.

Timothy's mother reported that he was reluctant to try new activities. During the assessment process, it was noted that Timothy tried new activities when offered, but had difficulty developing activities, making choices and initiating. This discovery provided useful information for his family, assuring them that they could expose Timothy to new experiences with confidence.

Upon assessing the musicality domain, it became clear to the music therapist that Timothy did not have an organized internal rhythm. This was evident by his difficulty altering his playing to match the therapist's rhythmic changes. He demonstrated a rigidity when playing rhythmic instruments, specifically playing a "drum roll" type rhythm on the instruments. It became clear to the music therapist that future therapy sessions would center on developing variety in Timothy's playing by creating structured activities to encourage him to explore different ways of playing the instruments. In addition, the musicality domain coupled with the social domain informed the therapist that Timothy had little to no awareness of mutual music making as he seemed to be playing simply to make noise as opposed to interactive music making. This, too, would be an area to develop in future sessions by creating situations for interaction to be required for successful music making.

The final numerical scoring of the IMTAP presented a clear picture of Timothy's level of functioning in the assessed domains. As shown in Table 7.1, Timothy's scores indicated areas of strength in expressive communication and social functioning. Timothy scored lowest in the musicality domain, followed closely by the social, fine motor, and receptive communication/auditory perception domains.

Table 7.1 Timothy's scores

Domain profile	Scores
Fine motor	36.6
Receptive communication/auditory perception	37.5
Expressive communication	83.2
Cognitive	57.6
Social	70.9
Emotional	35.4
Musicality	17.4
Sub-domain profile	
Fine motor	
A. Fundamentals	97.4
B. Strumming	51.9
C. Autoharp/Q Chord	13.3
D. Guitar/dulcimer	0
E. Piano	14.6
F. Pitched percussive/mallet	36.8
Domain total	**36.6**
Receptive communication/auditory perception	
A. Fundamentals	68.8
B. Direction following	81.8
C. Musical changes	10.0
D. Singing/vocalization	33.3
E. Rhythm	41.7
Domain total	**37.5**

continued on next page

Table 7.1 continued

Expressive communication	
A. Fundamentals	73.7
B. Non-vocal communication	N/A
C. Vocalizations	82.4
D. Spontaneous vocalizations	88.9
E. Verbalizations	100.0
F. Relational communication	69.6
G. Vocal idiosyncrasies	94.7
Domain total	**83.2**
Cognitive	
A. Fundamentals	90.0
B. Decision making	50.0
C. Direction following	90.9
D. Short-term recall/sequencing	81.8
E. Long-term recall	38.1
F. Academics	N/A
Domain total	**57.6**
Sensory	
A. Fundamentals	100.0
B. Tactile	100.0
C. Proprioceptive	100.0
D. Vestibular	100.0
E. Visual	95.5
F. Auditory	84.0
Domain total	**95.7**

Table 7.1 continued

Social	
A. Fundamentals	79.4
B. Participation	61.8
C. Turn-taking	66.7
D. Attention	76.9
E. Direction following	81.8
F. Relationship skills	56.3
Domain total	**70.9**
Emotional	
A. Affect	62.5
B. Differentiation/expression	15.0
C. Regulation	76.2
D. Self-awareness	13.3
Domain total	**35.4**
Musicality	
A. Fundamentals	75.0
B. Tempo	18.6
C. Rhythm	22.2
D. Dynamics	15.6
E. Vocal	21.0
F. Perfect and relative pitch	0.0
G. Creativity and development of musical ideas	4.4
H. Music reading	0.0
I. Accompaniment	20.0
Domain total	**17.4**

> **Therapeutic Goals for Timothy**
>
> - Develop self-awareness
> - Improve emotional expression
> - Improve creative expression and idea development
> - Improve relationship skills
> - Improve initiation skills
> - Improve imitation skills

A closer look at these domains allowed for the therapist to create a focused therapeutic plan. The sub-domain of social: self-awareness was identified as a need with a score of 13.3 and included in the goals for this client. Also in the social functioning area, the sub-domain of differentiation/expression scored a full 47.5 percentage points below the next highest sub-domain (affect). In parallel, the sub-domain of musicality: creativity and development of musical ideas resulted in the lowest score (4.4) of the scored sub-domains for this area. As a result, the realms of emotional and creative expression were included in the goals.

In the social domain, "relationship skills" was identified as scoring much lower in comparison to other sub-domains of the same area and added to the goal set. Lastly, to address the receptive communication/auditory perception domain, the specific areas of initiation and imitation were included as primary goals.

These goal areas were discussed with Timothy's parents as were the implications from administering the IMTAP. The scoring sheets provided an accessible tool for communicating the results to Timothy's parents, who were pleased with the thoroughness of the evaluation. The IMTAP was user-friendly and convenient for the therapist and provided an excellent measurement of Timothy's baseline skills as well as resources for development of future activities and interventions.

Chapter 8

The IMTAP Software and CD-ROM

The accompanying CD-ROM contains PDF files of all IMTAP forms as well as the IMTAP software, a fully automated system of client management, data collection, and assessment scoring. To access and print the IMTAP forms, go to the "IMTAP_Forms" folder of the CD-ROM.

Installing the IMTAP software

Important note: Do not move the IMTAP file folders from the location where they have been installed. To do so will prevent the program from operating correctly.

System requirements

- *Windows.* Pentium III 500 MHz or higher; 256MB of RAM; CD or DVD drive; SVGA (800 x 600) or higher resolution video adapter and display; Windows 2000 (Service Pack 4), Windows XP (Service Pack 2) or Windows Vista.
- *Mac OS X.* Macintosh computer with PowerPC G3, G4, or G5 processor; Macintosh computer with Intel-based processor; 256MB of RAM; CD or DVD drive; MAC OS X 10.3.9 for PowerPC processors; 10.4.5 for Intel-based processors.

Installing on a Windows system

1. On the CD-ROM, double click the "WINDOWS" folder.
2. Double click on "IMTAPv1_3.exe."

3. Select "Unzip" in the Win Zip Extractor window.

4. When the file has completed the extraction process, click "OK."

5. "Close" the Win Zip window.

6. Go to "Start" and "My Computer" to open a Windows Explorer window.

7. Go to the "C" drive on your computer.

8. Double-click the "IMTAPv1_3" folder.

9. Drag the "Shortcut to IMTAPv1_3" to your desktop.

10. You can now double-click the "Shortcut to IMTAPv1_3" icon on your desktop to open the program.

Installing on a Macintosh system

1. On the CD-ROM, double-click the "MAC_OS" folder.

2. Drag the file named "IMTAPv1_3.sitx" to your desktop.

3. Double-click the file to unstuff the contents.

4. After the unstuff operation is complete, an "IMTAPv1_3" folder will be on your desktop.

5. Within this folder, you may double-click on the "IMTAPv1_3" file to run the program. (*Note:* The file named "IMTAP_2007_v1_3.USR" is a system file and will not open the IMTAP program.)

   a. You may wish to create an alias of the "IMTAPv1_3" file and drag this alias to your desktop.

Important note: Do not move the IMTAP file folders from the location where they have been installed. To do so will prevent the program from operating correctly.

Using the IMTAP software

Carefully read Chapter 4 entitled "Administration Instructions" before beginning the assessment process.

1. Double-click on the IMTAP icon to open the program.

2. After reading the User Agreement, click on "I Agree" or "I Decline" located at the bottom of the User Agreement text.

3. After agreeing to the User Agreement, the IMTAP startup menu will be shown. From this menu, the two main hubs of the IMTAP software can be accessed, "Client Management" and "Report Menu."

4. Before beginning to use the software, a client record must be entered. See "Entering client records" below.

    Note: Information entered into the IMTAP software is dynamically saved. Unlike with a document, the user does not need to save the information. Any changes are saved automatically.

Entering client records

1. From the startup menu select "Client Management." This screen may also be accessed by selecting "Clients/Contact Info" from within the software.

2. On the upper left-hand portion of the Client Management screen, select "New."

3. Enter the client information in the spaces provided, using the tab key or the mouse to move between fields.

    Note: Enter all dates in the same format as your system allows for using numbers and slashes, i.e., mm/dd/yyyy for USA and dd/mm/yyyy for UK. Chronological ages will compute based on the entry of these dates.

Viewing and printing client records

1. To find a particular client click "Find" on the main Client Management screen.

2. Type the information identifying the client into the appropriate field and then hit the "Enter" key on your keyboard. For example, if you are looking for "Sue Smith," type "Sue" into the first name field. Searches can also be conducted by last name, date of birth, diagnosis, or any field on this screen. When searching for records, using the least amount of information will provide the most results. For example, if you enter "S" in the first name field you will get a list of all clients with "S" in their name (Stephen, Sue, Ross, etc.)

3. Searches resulting in multiple clients will be displayed in the list view. Select the client you wish to view by clicking anywhere on their name.

4. To view a list of all clients, select the "List View" tab on the Client Management screen. Clicking on any single client will direct you back to the main Client Management screen.

Exporting contact information

1. From the IMTAP Client Management screen click on "List View."

2. Click "Export Contacts" in the menu bar.

3. You are instructed to indicate the file location, name and type for your exported information. Click "OK" to continue or "Cancel" to stop.

4. After indicating the file location and name in the pop-up window, select the type of file you would like to export to, using the drop down list at the bottom of the window.

5. You will be given a choice to change the fields that will be exported and their order. This window is set to export all of the client contact information, including full names, phone numbers and addresses. You may wish to remove some of these choices if they are not needed. For example, you may not need to include phone numbers if you are using the export process to create mailing labels.

6. Click "Export."

7. Your new export file of the name and location you have designated is now created.

Conducting a client intake

1. From the Client Management screen, click "Intake" in the menu bar.

2. Enter the intake date when prompted.
   Note: Enter all dates in the same format as your system allows for using numbers and slashes, i.e., mm/dd/yyyy for USA and dd/mm/yyyy for UK. Chronological ages will compute based on the entry of these dates.

3. Enter the Interviewee name and Relationship to the Client in the appropriate fields.

4. Navigate through the various sections of the intake by clicking on the tabs for each domain. Within each tab is a list of questions to ask the interviewee. Indicate the responses by clicking on the "Yes" or "No" circle to the right of each question. A space is also provided to enter notes or further information for each question.

5. When clicking on the domain tabs, any completed domains will change to read "Done" when all questions for that domain have been answered.

6. Once all domains are complete, click on "Next Step >>."

   Note: The intake may only be conducted once and may not be altered once it is complete.

7. On the Intake Notes screen, enter notes or further comments from the interviewee as well as therapist impressions or comments.

8. Click on "Next >>."

9. Domain suggestions have now been created according to the intake data that was collected.

Recording assessment data

1. New assessments may be created in three ways:

   - Directly after completion of the intake, from the Domain Suggestions screen, click on "Begin Assessment >>."

   - From the main Client Management screen, click on "Assessment" in the menu bar.

   - From the Report Menu.
     - Click on the client name.
     - Click on "Assessment."
     - Click on "Begin New Assessment."

2. Enter the assessment date.

   Note: Enter all dates in the same format as your system allows for using numbers and slashes, i.e., mm/dd/yyyy for USA and dd/mm/yyyy for UK. Chronological ages will compute based on the entry of these dates.

3. If applicable, enter any additional assessment dates and whether the sessions were recorded.

4. On the Assessment Set Up screen, click on "Include" to add the appropriate domains to the assessment.

   Note: The musicality domain is always suggested. A domain does not have to be suggested to be included in the assessment. Domains that are not suggested may be included in the assessment.

5. After selecting the domains to be included, click on "Score Assessment >>."

6. The Assessment Overview screen lists the selected domains. The domains may be edited by clicking on "<< Return to Domain Selection/Assessment Setup," and clicking "Remove" or "Include" as necessary.

7. From the Assessment Overview screen, click on "Score Domain" to begin scoring.

8. Navigate through the various sub-domains of the domain by clicking on the tabs. Within each tab is a list of skills. Indicate client scores by clicking on "N," "R," "I," or "C" as appropriate.

9. Click on "Activities/Notes" to enter names of songs, activities, or instruments or to clarify client responses and preferences.

10. Click on "Sub-Domain Not Assessed" for sub-domains which were not assessed due to lack of time or resources.

    Note: "Sub-Domain Not Assessed" should be used only for sub-domains for which there was not time or sufficient resources to assess. For example, Fine Motor E (Piano) may be indicated as not assessed if a piano was not available. "Sub-Domain Not Assessed" should not be used if the sub-domain was not assessed due to client functioning level. For more information on how to score particular skills or sub-domains not assessed due to client functioning level, refer to Chapter 4, "Administration Instructions."

11. When clicking on the sub-domain tabs, completed sub-domains will change to read "Done" when all skills in that sub-domain have been scored.

12. When all sub-domains are scored (or labeled as "not assessed") click on "Domain Complete."

13. Repeat steps 7 through 12 for all domains to be assessed.

14. Once all domains are complete, click on "Assessment Complete/View Results >>."

15. If the assessment has included any cross-domain skills (skills which are included in more than one domain) those skills may be viewed now. Some points to consider in viewing cross-domain skills include:

    - If a cross-domain skill is scored more than once in the same assessment, are they scored the same?

    - If a cross-domain skill has been scored only once and scored as Never or Rarely, should the corresponding domain also be assessed? For example, if "Adapts playing to match tempo changes" is scored as Never in the musicality: tempo sub-domain, the therapist may be cued to also assess the corresponding sub-domain of gross motor: perceptual/visual/psycho motor.

- Click on "Assessment Results >>."

16. A numerical score is displayed for each sub-domain and domain that was assessed. Please refer to Chapter 4 "Administration Instructions," for information on how to interpret and use these scores.

17. To see a graphical representation of assessment scores, click on "View Graphs."

18. To view detail on any graph, click on the graph area.

Goals and objectives

1. Goals and objectives may be created in two ways:
   - From the main Client Management screen, click on "Goals" in the menu bar.
   - From the Report Menu:
     - Click on the client name.
     - Click on "Goals and Objectives."

2. Type a goal in the space provided.

3. Use the checkboxes to indicate the corresponding domain(s).

4. Enter a target date for the goal.

5. Type an objective for the goal in the space provided.

6. Enter a target date for the objective.

7. Continue entering objectives as needed by clicking in the next empty gray field under Objectives.

8. Click the navigation and control buttons to write, delete, view, or navigate through goals.

9. Click "Clients/Contact Info" or "Report Menu" in the menu bar to leave the goals and objectives screen.

   Note: You are required to enter at least one objective for each goal. If you do not wish to do so, you must delete the goal before leaving the screen.

The Report Menu

Use the Report Menu to view, edit, and create new assessments. Follow the on-screen instructions to access information and analyze assessment data.

Printing

Access printing and viewing controls through the Report Menu or in the menu bar of various screens.

Technical support

Support and contact information is listed in the About menu of the main menu bar. For technical support, email info@imtap.com.

USER WARNING: This database solution contains password(s) that can only be provided by the developer.

USER WARNING: This file is not customizable. Contact the developer for information on customizing this database solution.

Appendix A

IMTAP Forms

Intake Form
Cover Sheet
Session Outline
Domain Forms
    Gross Motor (GM)
    Fine Motor (FM)
    Oral Motor (OM)
    Sensory (SEN)
    Receptive Communication/Auditory Perception (RC)
    Expressive Communication (EC)
    Cognitive (COG)
    Emotional (EMO)
    Social (SOC)
    Musicality (MUS)
Summary Form
Goals and Objectives
Graph Form
Quantification Form

Individualized Music Therapy Assessment Profile (IMTAP)
Intake Form

Intake Date: _____
                                            Year   Month   Day

Client's Name: _____   Sex: M F   Birth Date: _____
                                                                                Year   Month   Day

Therapist's Name: _____   Chronological Age: _____
                                                                                   Years Months Days

Referring Individual: _____

Interviewee's Name: _____   Relationship to Client: _____

Please note: Questions on this form are of a personal and confidential nature. Therapist should exercise appropriate judgment when completing intake. Completion of this form is not a requirement for music therapy services.

General Information		
Does the child have a current diagnosis? *Dx:* Who gave this diagnosis?	Yes	No
Is the child on any medications? *Meds:*	Yes	No
Does the child have any allergies or sensitivities?	Yes	No
Are there any precautions I should take in working with the child? (i.e. seizures, biting, self-injurious behavior, etc.)	Yes	No
Does the child participate in any other therapies? *Therapies:*	Yes	No
Has the child had any previous musical experience or exposure?	Yes	No
Do you believe the child has any particular musical aptitude?	Yes	No
Are there any musicians in the child's immediate family? *Who?*	Yes	No
Have you noticed that the child has any musical preferences?	Yes	No
What benefit do you anticipate from music therapy?		

Copyright © Holly Tuesday Baxter, Julie Allis Berghofer, Lesa MacEwan, Judy Nelson, Kasi Peters, and Penny Roberts 2007

Client Name: _____ **Intake Date:** _____

Note to therapist: Any indications in the left-hand/shaded column indicate that this area of functioning should be assessed.

Gross Motor		
Have you noticed that the child has any gross motor difficulties?	Yes	No
Is the child fully ambulatory?	No	Yes
Does the child require any physical assistance?	Yes	No
Does the child have full use of all of his/her limbs?	No	Yes

Fine Motor		
Have you noticed that the child has any fine motor difficulties?	Yes	No
Is the child able to perform fine motor tasks with both hands? (i.e. eat with utensils, button a button, hold a pencil)	No	Yes
Does the child frequently drop items or have difficulty holding objects?	Yes	No

Oral		
Does the child have any feeding issues?	Yes	No
Does the child have any respiratory issues?	Yes	No

Sensory		
Have you noticed that the child has any sensory issues?	Yes	No
Does the child resist physical support?	Yes	No
Does the child engage in any repetitive behaviors?	Yes	No
Does the child have any deficits in hearing, vision, or other senses?	Yes	No
Does the child have any sensitivities to or extreme preferences for particular sounds?	Yes	No
Is the child over-stimulated by sounds, lights, or crowds?	Yes	No

Copyright © Holly Tuesday Baxter, Julie Allis Berghofer, Lesa MacEwan, Judy Nelson, Kasi Peters, and Penny Roberts 2007

Client Name: _____ **Intake Date:** _____

Receptive Communication/Auditory Perception		
Has the child been diagnosed with any hearing difficulties? *If so, has an audiogram been done and what were results:*	Yes	No
Does the child have difficulty hearing sounds or understanding speech?	Yes	No
Does the child have a history of ear infections?	Yes	No
Does the child understand or react to what is being said to him/her?	No	Yes

Expressive Communication		
Have you noticed that the child has any speech or language difficulties?	Yes	No
Does the child communicate verbally? *If not, please indicate mode of communication:*	No	Yes
Do others easily understand the child?	No	Yes
Does the child have any idiosyncratic speech?	Yes	No

Cognitive		
Have you noticed that the child has any cognitive deficits or difficulties?	Yes	No
Does the child have an IEP (Individualized Education Plan)?	Yes	No
Is the child in with same-age peers in their educational setting?	No	Yes

Emotional		
Have you noticed that the child has any emotional difficulties?	Yes	No
Does the child show emotions appropriately?	No	Yes
Does the child tantrum or get angry easily?	Yes	No
Has the child suffered any emotional trauma or recent change in life circumstances?	Yes	No

Copyright © Holly Tuesday Baxter, Julie Allis Berghofer, Lesa MacEwan, Judy Nelson, Kasi Peters, and Penny Roberts 2007

Client Name: _____ **Intake Date:** _____

Social		
Have you noticed that the child has any social difficulties?	Yes	No
Does the child have any difficulty relating to family members?	Yes	No
Does the child have a social group of like-aged peers?	No	Yes
Does the child participate in conversation or play with others?	No	Yes
Does the child have any particular difficulties in school or other social situations?	Yes	No

Is there anything we have not covered that you feel is important?

_____

_____

_____

_____

_____

Therapist notes:

_____

_____

_____

_____

_____

Copyright © Holly Tuesday Baxter, Julie Allis Berghofer, Lesa MacEwan, Judy Nelson, Kasi Peters, and Penny Roberts 2007

Client Name: _____ **Intake Date:** _____

Intake Summary:

Please check applicable categories based on above information:

- ☐ Gross Motor
- ☐ Fine Motor
- ☐ Oral Motor
- ☐ Sensory
- ☐ Receptive Communication/Auditory Perception
- ☐ Expressive Communication
- ☐ Cognitive
- ☐ Emotional
- ☐ Social
- ☒ Musicality

_____   _____
Signature   Date

Individualized Music Therapy Assessment Profile (IMTAP)
Cover Sheet

Intake Date: _____
Year   Month   Day

Client's Name: _____ Sex: M F   Birth Date: _____
Year   Month   Day

Therapist's Name: _____ Chronological Age: _____
Years   Months   Days

Additional Assessment Date(s): _____ Date to be Reviewed: _____

Videotaped: ____ Yes ____ No

Domains to be assessed (please check):

- ☐ Gross Motor
- ☐ Fine Motor
- ☐ Oral Motor
- ☐ Sensory
- ☐ Receptive Communication/Auditory Perception
- ☐ Expressive Communication
- ☐ Cognitive
- ☐ Emotional
- ☐ Social
- ☒ Musicality

Please use the following guidelines to assist in the assessment process:
1. Assessment to be completed in 1–3 individual MT sessions by the same therapist.
2. Assessment to be recorded on video when possible.
3. Activities, music, instruments, techniques used to be indicated in each category.
4. Multiple responses may be assessed within one activity.

Rating
N = Never = 0%
R = Rarely = Under 50%
I = Inconsistent = 50–79%
C = Consistent = 80–100%

Copyright © Holly Tuesday Baxter, Julie Allis Berghofer, Lesa MacEwan, Judy Nelson, Kasi Peters, and Penny Roberts 2007

Individualized Music Therapy Assessment Profile (IMTAP)
Session Outline

Client: _____ D.O.B./Age: _____

Date(s) of Assessment: _____

Assessment Conducted By: _____

Categories to be assessed (please check):

- ☐ Gross Motor activities

- ☐ Fine Motor activities

- ☐ Oral Motor activities

- ☐ Sensory activities

- ☐ Receptive Communication/Auditory Perception activities

- ☐ Expressive Communication activities

- ☐ Cognitive activities

- ☐ Emotional activities

- ☐ Social activities

- ☒ Musicality activities

Copyright © Holly Tuesday Baxter, Julie Allis Berghofer, Lesa MacEwan, Judy Nelson, Kasi Peters, and Penny Roberts 2007

IMTAP - Gross Motor

Client Name: _____   **Assessment Date(s):** _____

Rating Scale:
N = Never = 0%   R = Rarely = Under 50%   I = Inconsistent = 50–79%   C = Consistent = 80–100%

A. Fundamentals

i.	Moves spontaneously	N_0	R_1	I_2	C_3		
ii.	Displays appropriate muscle tone during movement	N_0	R_1	I_2	C_3		
iii.	Reaches to touch/play instrument	N_0	R_1	I_2	C_3		
iv.	Displays heel-toe gait	N_0	R_1	I_2	C_3		
v.	Displays even walking gait		N_0	R_2	I_3	C_4	
vi.	Established left/right dominance		N_0	R_2	I_3	C_4	
vii.	Crosses body midline		N_0	R_2	I_3	C_4	
viii.	Coordinates playing of two different instruments		N_0	R_2	I_3	C_4	
	Column Totals:						
	Add Column Totals to calculate Raw Score:						

Activities/Notes

B. Perceptual/Visual/Psycho Motor   n/a ☐

i.	Demonstrates motor agitation (tremor) – *note reversed grading scale*	C_0	I_1	R_2	N_3		
ii.	Unconscious body movements in tempo CD	N_0	R_1	I_2	C_3		
iii.	Conscious body movement in tempo CD	N_0	R_1	I_2	C_3		
iv.	Moves in organized manner	N_0	R_1	I_2	C_3		
v.	Movements are related to musical stimuli	N_0	R_1	I_2	C_3		
vi.	Plays in tempo of therapist 1–4 measures CD		N_0	R_2	I_3	C_4	
vii.	Imitates gross motor movements of therapist		N_0	R_2	I_3	C_4	
viii.	Demonstrates ability to stop/go on cue		N_0	R_2	I_3	C_4	
ix.	Adapts playing in response to non-musical cues		N_0	R_2	I_3	C_4	
x.	Adapts playing to match dynamic changes		N_0	R_2	I_3	C_4	
xi.	Adapts playing to match tempo changes CD		N_0	R_2	I_3	C_4	
xii.	Demonstrates ability to sequence 2 movements		N_0	R_2	I_3	C_4	

Copyright © Holly Tuesday Baxter, Julie Allis Berghofer, Lesa MacEwan, Judy Nelson, Kasi Peters, and Penny Roberts 2007

IMTAP - Gross Motor

Client Name: _____   **Assessment Date(s):** _____

Rating Scale:
N = Never = 0%   R = Rarely = Under 50%   I = Inconsistent = 50–79%   C = Consistent = 80–100%

B. Perceptual/Visual/Psycho Motor (continued)							
xiii. Demonstrates ability to sequence 3 or more movements				N_0	R_3	I_4	C_5
xiv. Adapts playing to match meter changes *CD*				N_0	R_4	I_5	C_6
xv. Demonstrates ability to develop movement sequences				N_0	R_4	I_5	C_6
Column Totals:							
Add Column Totals to calculate Raw Score:							

Activities/Notes

Summary

Sub-Domain	n/a	Raw Score		Possible		Final Score
A. Fundamentals			÷	28	=	%
B. Perceptual/Visual/Psycho Motor			÷	60	=	%
Domain Total (Gross Motor)			÷		=	%

CD = Cross Domain Skills

IMTAP - Fine Motor

Client Name: _____   **Assessment Date(s):** _____

Rating Scale:
N = Never = 0%   R = Rarely = Under 50%   I = Inconsistent = 50–79%   C = Consistent = 80–100%

A. Fundamentals

i.	Displays use of both hands	N_0	R_1	I_2	C_3		
ii.	Uses palmar grasp	N_0	R_1	I_2	C_3		
iii.	Uses pincer grasp	N_0	R_1	I_2	C_3		
iv.	Holds object/instrument independently with one hand	N_0	R_1	I_2	C_3		
v.	Holds object/instrument independently with two hands	N_0	R_1	I_2	C_3		
vi.	Established left/right hand dominance		N_0	R_2	I_3	C_4	
vii.	Forms shapes with fingers and/or isolates fingers during finger play activities		N_0	R_2	I_3	C_4	
viii.	Plays instrument with alternating hands		N_0	R_2	I_3	C_4	
ix.	Sustains palmar grasp with dominant hand		N_0	R_2	I_3	C_4	
x.	Sustains palmar grasp with non-dominant hand		N_0	R_2	I_3	C_4	
xi.	Organizes alternating hands in playing		N_0	R_2	I_3	C_4	
	Column Totals:						
	Add Column Totals to calculate Raw Score:						

Activities/Notes

B. Strumming   n/a ☐

i.	Whole hand	N_0	R_1	I_2	C_3		
ii.	Single finger	N_0	R_1	I_2	C_3		
iii.	Whole hand with pulse			N_0	R_3	I_4	C_5
iv.	Single finger with pulse			N_0	R_3	I_4	C_5
v.	Strums with pick			N_0	R_3	I_4	C_5
vi.	Strums with pick and pulse				N_0	R_4	I_5	C_6
	Column Totals:						
	Add Column Totals to calculate Raw Score:						

Activities/Notes

Copyright © Holly Tuesday Baxter, Julie Allis Berghofer, Lesa MacEwan, Judy Nelson, Kasi Peters, and Penny Roberts 2007

IMTAP - Fine Motor

Client Name: _____   **Assessment Date(s):** _____

Rating Scale:
N = Never = 0%   R = Rarely = Under 50%   I = Inconsistent = 50–79%   C = Consistent = 80–100%

C. Autoharp/Q Chord   n/a ☐

i.	Explores chord buttons	N_0	R_1	I_2	C_3		
ii.	Depresses single button on cue	N_0	R_1	I_2	C_3		
iii.	Coordinates press and strum		N_0	R_2	I_3	C_4	
iv.	Plays simple accompaniment using chord chart $_{CD}$			N_0	R_3	I_4	C_5
	Column Totals:						
	Add Column Totals to calculate **Raw Score**:						

Activities/Notes

D. Guitar/Dulcimer   n/a ☐

i.	Forms chords with prompting				N_0	R_4	I_5	C_6
ii.	Approximates simple chord positions				N_0	R_4	I_5	C_6
iii.	Forms chords in simple musical pattern				N_0	R_4	I_5	C_6
iv.	Forms chords in advanced musical pattern				N_0	R_4	I_5	C_6
v.	Plays using chord chart				N_0	R_4	I_5	C_6
vi.	Plays individual strings				N_0	R_4	I_5	C_6
vii.	Plays individual strings with pulse				N_0	R_4	I_5	C_6
	Column Totals:						
	Add Column Totals to calculate **Raw Score**:						

Activities/Notes

E. Piano   n/a ☐

i.	Coordinates both hands	N_0	R_1	I_2	C_3		
ii.	Uses fingers of dominant hand without splaying	N_0	R_1	I_2	C_3		
iii.	Uses fingers of non-dominant hand without splaying	N_0	R_1	I_2	C_3		
iv.	Uses single finger of dominant hand		N_0	R_2	I_3	C_4	
v.	Uses single finger of non-dominant hand		N_0	R_2	I_3	C_4	
vi.	Sequences multiple fingers on dominant hand				N_0	R_4	I_5	C_6
vii.	Sequences multiple fingers on non-dominant hand				N_0	R_4	I_5	C_6

Copyright © Holly Tuesday Baxter, Julie Allis Berghofer, Lesa MacEwan, Judy Nelson, Kasi Peters, and Penny Roberts 2007

IMTAP - Fine Motor

Client Name: _____   **Assessment Date(s):** _____

Rating Scale:
N = Never = 0%   R = Rarely = Under 50%   I = Inconsistent = 50–79%   C = Consistent = 80–100%

E. Piano (continued)							
viii. Forms triads with dominant hand				N_0	R_4	I_5	C_6
ix. Forms triads with non-dominant hand				N_0	R_4	I_5	C_6
Column Totals:							
Add Column Totals to calculate Raw Score:							

Activities/Notes

F. Pitched Percussive/Mallet							n/a ☐
i. Plays small instrument with mallet when presented	N_0	R_1	I_2	C_3			
ii. Plays isolated note with mallet from multiple choices		N_0	R_2	I_3	C_4		
iii. Plays mallet with strike and retract motion		N_0	R_2	I_3	C_4		
iv. Sequences simple pattern of notes			N_0	R_3	I_4	C_5	
Column Totals:							
Add Column Totals to calculate Raw Score:							

Activities/Notes

Summary

Sub-Domain	n/a	Raw Score		Possible		Final Score
A. Fundamentals			÷	39	=	%
B. Strumming			÷	27	=	%
C. Autoharp/Q Chord			÷	15	=	%
D. Guitar/Dulcimer			÷	42	=	%
E. Piano			÷	41	=	%
F. Pitched Percussive/Mallet			÷	19	=	%
Domain Total (Fine Motor)			÷		=	%

CD = Cross Domain Skills

IMTAP - Oral Motor

Client Name: _____   **Assessment Date(s):** _____

Rating Scale:
N = Never = 0%   R = Rarely = Under 50%   I = Inconsistent = 50–79%   C = Consistent = 80–100%

A. Fundamentals

i.	Demonstrates full range of motion when opening	N_0	R_1	I_2	C_3		
ii.	Demonstrates full range of motion when smiling	N_0	R_1	I_2	C_3		
iii.	Demonstrates full range of motion when puckering	N_0	R_1	I_2	C_3		
iv.	Attains full mouth closure	N_0	R_1	I_2	C_3		
	Column Totals:						
	Add Column Totals to calculate Raw Score:						

Activities/Notes

B. Air Production   n/a ☐

i.	Tolerates putting mouthpiece to lips CD	N_0	R_1	I_2	C_3		
ii.	Produces tone	N_0	R_1	I_2	C_3		
iii.	Able to produce tone on cue		N_0	R_2	I_3	C_4	
iv.	Produces tone of one second or less		N_0	R_2	I_3	C_4	
v.	Produces tone of greater than one second		N_0	R_2	I_3	C_4	
vi.	Produces simple rhythmic pattern		N_0	R_2	I_3	C_4	
vii.	Integrates tone production and gross motor movement		N_0	R_2	I_3	C_4	
viii.	Integrates tone production and fine motor movement		N_0	R_2	I_3	C_4	
	Column Totals:						
	Add Column Totals to calculate Raw Score:						

Activities/Notes

Copyright © Holly Tuesday Baxter, Julie Allis Berghofer, Lesa MacEwan, Judy Nelson, Kasi Peters, and Penny Roberts 2007

IMTAP - Oral Motor

Client Name: _____ **Assessment Date(s):** _____

Summary

Sub-Domain	n/a	Raw Score		Possible		Final Score
A. Fundamentals	▓		÷	12	=	%
B. Air Production			÷	30	=	%
Domain Total (Oral Motor)			÷		=	%

CD = Cross Domain Skills

Copyright © Holly Tuesday Baxter, Julie Allis Berghofer, Lesa MacEwan, Judy Nelson, Kasi Peters, and Penny Roberts 2007

IMTAP - Sensory

Client Name: _____   **Assessment Date(s):** _____

Rating Scale:
N = Never = 0%   R = Rarely = Under 50%   I = Inconsistent = 50–79%   C = Consistent = 80–100%

A. Fundamentals

i.	Integrates sensory input of two types	N_0	R_1	I_2	C_3		
ii.	Integrates multiple sensory input types	N_0	R_1	I_2	C_3		
	Column Totals:						
	Add Column Totals to calculate Raw Score:						

Activities/Notes

B. Tactile   n/a ☐

i.	Seeks firm pressure	C_0	I_1	R_2	N_3		
ii.	Seeks light pressure	C_0	I_1	R_2	N_3		
iii.	Tolerates firm pressure	N_0	R_1	I_2	C_3		
iv.	Tolerates light pressure	N_0	R_1	I_2	C_3		
v.	Tolerates lightweight manipulatives	N_0	R_1	I_2	C_3		
vi.	Tolerates putting mouthpiece to lips CD	N_0	R_1	I_2	C_3		
vii.	Demonstrates ability to begin/stop tactile activity	N_0	R_1	I_2	C_3		
viii.	Demonstrates awareness of or attends to tactile input	N_0	R_1	I_2	C_3		
ix.	Remains physically open when instrument presented	N_0	R_1	I_2	C_3		
x.	Sustains grasp of instrument or mallet for four seconds or more	N_0	R_1	I_2	C_3		
xi.	Uses open hand on instruments	N_0	R_1	I_2	C_3		
	Column Totals:						
	Add Column Totals to calculate Raw Score:						

Activities/Notes

C. Proprioceptive   n/a ☐

i.	Seeks proprioceptive input	C_0	I_1	R_2	N_3		
ii.	Tolerates proprioceptive input	N_0	R_1	I_2	C_3		

Copyright © Holly Tuesday Baxter, Julie Allis Berghofer, Lesa MacEwan, Judy Nelson, Kasi Peters, and Penny Roberts 2007

IMTAP - Sensory

Client Name: _____   **Assessment Date(s):** _____

Rating Scale:
N = Never = 0%   R = Rarely = Under 50%   I = Inconsistent = 50–79%   C = Consistent = 80–100%

C. Proprioceptive (continued)							
iii. Demonstrates ability to begin/stop proprioceptive activity	N_0	R_1	I_2	C_3			
iv. Integrates proprioceptive tasks into activities		N_0	R_2	I_3	C_4		
Column Totals:							
Add Column Totals to calculate Raw Score:							
Activities/Notes							

D. Vestibular							n/a ☐
i. Seeks vestibular input	C_0	I_1	R_2	N_3			
ii. Tolerates vestibular input	N_0	R_1	I_2	C_3			
iii. Demonstrates ability to begin/stop vestibular activity	N_0	R_1	I_2	C_3			
iv. Demonstrates ability to return to task after vestibular distraction with prompts	N_0	R_1	I_2	C_3			
v. Demonstrates ability to return to task after vestibular distraction without prompts		N_0	R_2	I_3	C_4		
Column Totals:							
Add Column Totals to calculate Raw Score:							
Activities/Notes							

E. Visual					n/a ☐
i. Seeks visual input	C_0	I_1	R_2	N_3	
ii. Tolerates visual input	N_0	R_1	I_2	C_3	
iii. Demonstrates ability to begin/stop visual activity	N_0	R_1	I_2	C_3	
iv. Demonstrates ability to return to task after visual distraction with prompts	N_0	R_1	I_2	C_3	
v. Demonstrates awareness of or attends to visual input	N_0	R_1	I_2	C_3	

Copyright © Holly Tuesday Baxter, Julie Allis Berghofer, Lesa MacEwan, Judy Nelson, Kasi Peters, and Penny Roberts 2007

IMTAP - Sensory

Client Name: _____   **Assessment Date(s):** _____

Rating Scale:
N = Never = 0%   R = Rarely = Under 50%   I = Inconsistent = 50–79%   C = Consistent = 80–100%

E. Visual (continued)							
vi.	Maintains gaze of object or person for appropriate length	N_0	R_1	I_2	C_3		
vii.	Demonstrates ability to return to task after visual distraction without prompts		N_0	R_2	I_3	C_4	
	Column Totals:						
	Add Column Totals to calculate *Raw Score*:						

Activities/Notes

F. Auditory								n/a ☐
i.	Seeks auditory input	C_0	I_1	R_2	N_3			
ii.	Demonstrates awareness of sound vs. silence *CD*	N_0	R_1	I_2	C_3			
iii.	Tolerates auditory input	N_0	R_1	I_2	C_3			
iv.	Tolerates a variety of sounds	N_0	R_1	I_2	C_3			
v.	Demonstrates ability to begin/stop auditory activity	N_0	R_1	I_2	C_3			
vi.	Demonstrates awareness of or attends to auditory input	N_0	R_1	I_2	C_3			
vii.	Demonstrates ability to return to task after auditory distraction with prompts	N_0	R_1	I_2	C_3			
viii.	Demonstrates ability to return to task after auditory distraction without prompts		N_0	R_2	I_3	C_4		
	Column Totals:							
	Add Column Totals to calculate *Raw Score*:							

Activities/Notes

Copyright © Holly Tuesday Baxter, Julie Allis Berghofer, Lesa MacEwan, Judy Nelson, Kasi Peters, and Penny Roberts 2007

IMTAP - Sensory

Client Name: _____ **Assessment Date(s):** _____

Summary

Sub-Domain	n/a	Raw Score	Possible			Final Score
A. Fundamentals	▓		÷	6	=	%
B. Tactile			÷	33	=	%
C. Proprioceptive			÷	13	=	%
D. Vestibular			÷	16	=	%
E. Visual			÷	22	=	%
F. Auditory			÷	25	=	%
Domain Total (Sensory)			÷		=	%

CD = Cross Domain Skills

Copyright © Holly Tuesday Baxter, Julie Allis Berghofer, Lesa MacEwan, Judy Nelson, Kasi Peters, and Penny Roberts 2007

IMTAP - Receptive Communication/Auditory Perception

Client Name: _____ **Assessment Date(s):** _____

Rating Scale:
N = Never = 0%   R = Rarely = Under 50%   I = Inconsistent = 50–79%   C = Consistent = 80–100%

A. Fundamentals

i.	Demonstrates awareness of sound vs. silence CD	N_0	R_1	I_2	C_3		
ii.	Turns head to sound source	N_0	R_1	I_2	C_3		
iii.	Localizes eye gaze to sound source	N_0	R_1	I_2	C_3		
iv.	Discriminates between two differing sounds	N_0	R_1	I_2	C_3		
v.	Imitates simple musical motif		N_0	R_2	I_3	C_4	
	Column Totals:						
	Add Column Totals to calculate *Raw Score*:						

Activities/Notes

B. Direction Following n/a ☐

i.	Follows one-step verbal direction CD	N_0	R_1	I_2	C_3		
ii.	Follows two-step verbal direction CD		N_0	R_2	I_3	C_4	
iii.	Follows simple musical cues CD		N_0	R_2	I_3	C_4	
	Column Totals:						
	Add Column Totals to calculate *Raw Score*:						

Activities/Notes

C. Musical Changes n/a ☐

i.	Demonstrates awareness of gross tempo changes	N_0	R_1	I_2	C_3		
ii.	Demonstrates awareness of gross pitch changes	N_0	R_1	I_2	C_3		
iii.	Demonstrates awareness of gross dynamic changes CD	N_0	R_1	I_2	C_3		
iv.	Demonstrates awareness of meter changes			N_0	R_3	I_4	C_5
v.	Demonstrates awareness of changes in intensity/mood			N_0	R_3	I_4	C_5

Copyright © Holly Tuesday Baxter, Julie Allis Berghofer, Lesa MacEwan, Judy Nelson, Kasi Peters, and Penny Roberts 2007

IMTAP - Receptive Communication/Auditory Perception

Client Name: _____   **Assessment Date(s):** _____

Rating Scale:
N = Never = 0%   R = Rarely = Under 50%   I = Inconsistent = 50–79%   C = Consistent = 80–100%

C. Musical Changes (continued)							n/a ☐
vi. Plays melodically in tonality of improvisation				N_0	R_3	I_4	C_5
vii. Plays in appropriate key without prompting					N_0	R_4	I_5	C_6
Column Totals:							
Add Column Totals to calculate Raw Score:							

Activities/Notes

D. Singing/Vocalizing							n/a ☐
i. Vocalizes in response to aural stimuli	N_0	R_1	I_2	C_3			
ii. Vocalizes in response to therapist speaking	N_0	R_1	I_2	C_3			
iii. Vocalizes in response to therapist singing	N_0	R_1	I_2	C_3			
iv. Vocalizes in response to un-pitched instruments	N_0	R_1	I_2	C_3			
v. Vocalizes in response to pitched instruments	N_0	R_1	I_2	C_3			
vi. Vocalizes in response to particular musical style/idiom CD	N_0	R_1	I_2	C_3			
vii. Unconscious vocalizations in tonality CD	N_0	R_1	I_2	C_3			
viii. Sings in key with therapist		N_0	R_2	I_3	C_4		
ix. Vocalizes in provided musical pause		N_0	R_2	I_3	C_4		
x. Imitates descending musical interval greater than M2		N_0	R_2	I_3	C_4		
xi. Imitates ascending musical interval greater than M2		N_0	R_2	I_3	C_4		
xii. Sings pitched melody accurately CD		N_0	R_2	I_3	C_4		
xiii. Imitates descending step-wise musical motifs			N_0	R_3	I_4	C_5	
xiv. Imitates ascending step-wise musical motifs			N_0	R_3	I_4	C_5	
Column Totals:							
Add Column Totals to calculate Raw Score:							

Activities/Notes

Copyright © Holly Tuesday Baxter, Julie Allis Berghofer, Lesa MacEwan, Judy Nelson, Kasi Peters, and Penny Roberts 2007

IMTAP - Receptive Communication/Auditory Perception

Client Name: _____   **Assessment Date(s):** _____

Rating Scale:
N = Never = 0%   R = Rarely = Under 50%   I = Inconsistent = 50–79%   C = Consistent = 80–100%

E. Rhythm						n/a ☐
i. Plays in tempo of therapist 1–4 measures CD		N_0	R_2	I_3	C_4	
ii. Imitates simple rhythmic pattern CD		N_0	R_2	I_3	C_4	
iii. Imitates intermediate rhythmic pattern CD		N_0	R_2	I_3	C_4	
Column Totals:						
Add Column Totals to calculate *Raw Score*:						

Activities/Notes

Summary

Sub-Domain	n/a	Raw Score	Possible		Final Score
A. Fundamentals			÷ 16	=	%
B. Direction Following			÷ 11	=	%
C. Musical Changes			÷ 30	=	%
D. Singing/Vocalizing			÷ 51	=	%
E. Rhythm			÷ 12	=	%
Domain Total (Receptive Communication/ Auditory Perception)			÷	=	%

CD = Cross Domain Skills

Copyright © Holly Tuesday Baxter, Julie Allis Berghofer, Lesa MacEwan, Judy Nelson, Kasi Peters, and Penny Roberts 2007

IMTAP - Expressive Communication

Client Name: _____   **Assessment Date(s):** _____

Rating Scale:
N = Never = 0%   R = Rarely = Under 50%   I = Inconsistent = 50–79%   C = Consistent = 80–100%

A. Fundamentals

i.	Attempts to communicate	N_0	R_1	I_2	C_3			
ii.	Communicates without frustration	N_0	R_1	I_2	C_3			
iii.	Communicates needs and desires	N_0	R_1	I_2	C_3			
iv.	Communicates ideas and concepts		N_0	R_2	I_3	C_4		
v.	Communicates emotional content or idea development				N_0	R_4	I_5	C_6
	Column Totals:							
	Add Column Totals to calculate Raw Score:							

Activities/Notes

B. Non-vocal Communication   n/a ☐
N/A if client's chosen mode of communication is vocal/verbal

i.	Leads or moves therapist as means of communication	N_0	R_1	I_2	C_3			
ii.	Gestures	N_0	R_1	I_2	C_3			
iii.	Combines gesture and leading/moving of therapist	N_0	R_1	I_2	C_3			
iv.	Combines gesture with vocalization	N_0	R_1	I_2	C_3			
	Column Totals:							
	Add Column Totals to calculate Raw Score:							

Activities/Notes

C. Vocalizations   n/a ☐
N/A if client's chosen mode of communication is non-vocal

i.	Vocalizations are of clear tonal quality	N_0	R_1	I_2	C_3
ii.	Vocalizations are of appropriate volume	N_0	R_1	I_2	C_3
iii.	Vocalizations are in moderate pitch range	N_0	R_1	I_2	C_3

Copyright © Holly Tuesday Baxter, Julie Allis Berghofer, Lesa MacEwan, Judy Nelson, Kasi Peters, and Penny Roberts 2007

IMTAP - Expressive Communication

Client Name: _____   **Assessment Date(s):** _____

Rating Scale:
N = Never = 0%   R = Rarely = Under 50%   I = Inconsistent = 50–79%   C = Consistent = 80–100%

C. Vocalizations – (continued)						
iv. Vocalizations are of phrase length		N_0	R_2	I_3	C_4	
v. Vocalizations are of sentence length		N_0	R_2	I_3	C_4	
Column Totals:						
Add Column Totals to calculate Raw Score:						

Activities/Notes

D. Spontaneous Vocalizations						n/a ☐
i. Vocalizes with therapist	N_0	R_1	I_2	C_3		
ii. Vocalizations are of non-imitative type	N_0	R_1	I_2	C_3		
iii. Vocalizations are purposefully imitative	N_0	R_1	I_2	C_3		
Column Totals:						
Add Column Totals to calculate Raw Score:						

Activities/Notes

E. Verbalizations						n/a ☐
N/A if client's chosen mode of communication is non-vocal						
i. Verbalizations are intelligible	N_0	R_1	I_2	C_3		
ii. Verbalizes single words	N_0	R_1	I_2	C_3		
iii. Verbalizations are of phrase length		N_0	R_2	I_3	C_4	
iv. Verbalizations are of sentence length		N_0	R_2	I_3	C_4	
Column Totals:						
Add Column Totals to calculate Raw Score:						

Activities/Notes

IMTAP - Expressive Communication

Client Name: _____   **Assessment Date(s):** _____

Rating Scale:
N = Never = 0%   R = Rarely = Under 50%   I = Inconsistent = 50–79%   C = Consistent = 80–100%

F. Relational Communication						n/a ☐
i. Answers closed (yes/no) questions CD	N_0	R_1	I_2	C_3		
ii. Answers binary questions		N_0	R_2	I_3	C_4	
iii. Participates in simple reciprocal conversation		N_0	R_2	I_3	C_4	
iv. Initiates conversation appropriate to situation		N_0	R_2	I_3	C_4	
v. Asks questions appropriately		N_0	R_2	I_3	C_4	
vi. Answers open questions		N_0	R_2	I_3	C_4	
Column Totals:						
Add Column Totals to calculate Raw Score:						

Activities/Notes

G. Vocal Idiosyncrasies						n/a ☐
Note reversal of grading scale through this section						
i. Vocalizations contain inflectional babble/jargon	C_0	I_1	R_2	N_3		
ii. Vocalizations are echolalic	C_0	I_1	R_2	N_3		
iii. Vocalizations are unconscious	C_0	I_1	R_2	N_3		
iv. Vocalizations are delayed	C_0	I_1	R_2	N_3		
v. Vocalizations are clipped or of irregular meter	C_0	I_1	R_2	N_3		
vi. Vocalizations are scripted		C_0	I_2	R_3	N_4	
Column Totals:						
Add Column Totals to calculate Raw Score:						

Activities/Notes

Copyright © Holly Tuesday Baxter, Julie Allis Berghofer, Lesa MacEwan, Judy Nelson, Kasi Peters, and Penny Roberts 2007

IMTAP - Expressive Communication

Client Name: _____   **Assessment Date(s):** _____

Summary

Sub-Domain	n/a	Raw Score	Possible			Final Score
A. Fundamentals	▓		÷	19	=	%
B. Non-vocal Communication			÷	12	=	%
C. Vocalizations			÷	17	=	%
D. Spontaneous Vocalizations			÷	9	=	%
E. Verbalizations			÷	14	=	%
F. Relational Communication			÷	23	=	%
G. Vocal Idiosyncrasies			÷	19	=	%
Domain Total (Expressive Communication)			÷		=	%

CD = Cross Domain Skills

Copyright © Holly Tuesday Baxter, Julie Allis Berghofer, Lesa MacEwan, Judy Nelson, Kasi Peters, and Penny Roberts 2007

IMTAP - Cognitive

Client Name: _____   **Assessment Date(s):** _____

Rating Scale:
N = Never = 0%   R = Rarely = Under 50%   I = Inconsistent = 50–79%   C = Consistent = 80–100%

A. Fundamentals

i.	Sustains activity length attention span CD	N_0	R_1	I_2	C_3		
ii.	Looks for hidden or dropped object	N_0	R_1	I_2	C_3		
iii.	Demonstrates understanding of rules and structures		N_0	R_2	I_3	C_4	

Column Totals:
Add Column Totals to calculate **Raw Score:**

Activities/Notes

B. Decision Making   n/a ☐

i.	Answers closed (yes/no) questions CD	N_0	R_1	I_2	C_3		
ii.	Makes choice between two presented concrete options	N_0	R_1	I_2	C_3		
iii.	Makes choice between three presented concrete options		N_0	R_2	I_3	C_4	
iv.	Answers abstract binary questions		N_0	R_2	I_3	C_4	
v.	Makes choice without prompting		N_0	R_2	I_3	C_4	

Column Totals:
Add Column Totals to calculate **Raw Score:**

Activities/Notes

Copyright © Holly Tuesday Baxter, Julie Allis Berghofer, Lesa MacEwan, Judy Nelson, Kasi Peters, and Penny Roberts 2007

IMTAP - Cognitive

Client Name: _____ **Assessment Date(s):** _____

<u>Rating Scale:</u>
N = Never = 0%   R = Rarely = Under 50%   I = Inconsistent = 50–79%   C = Consistent = 80–100%

C. Direction Following							n/a ☐
i. Follows one-step verbal direction CD		N_0	R_1	I_2	C_3		
ii. Follows two-step verbal direction CD			N_0	R_2	I_3	C_4	
iii. Follows simple musical cues CD			N_0	R_2	I_3	C_4	
Column Totals:							
Add Column Totals to calculate **Raw Score:**							

Activities/Notes

D. Short-term Recall/Sequencing							n/a ☐
i. Recalls new information within activity		N_0	R_1	I_2	C_3		
ii. Sequences two objects within activity		N_0	R_1	I_2	C_3		
iii. Sequences three objects within activity				N_0	R_3	I_4	C_5
Column Totals:							
Add Column Totals to calculate **Raw Score:**							

Activities/Notes

E. Long-term Recall							n/a ☐
Assessed only if client is seen for more than one session							
i. Recalls therapist's name		N_0	R_2	I_3	C_4		
ii. Recalls names of instruments		N_0	R_2	I_3	C_4		
iii. Recalls function of instruments		N_0	R_2	I_3	C_4		
iv. Demonstrates awareness of MT routine		N_0	R_2	I_3	C_4		
v. Requests previously presented activities/songs		N_0	R_2	I_3	C_4		
vi. Sings correct lyrics without visual/aural cues			N_0	R_3	I_4	C_5	
vii. Plays simple accompaniment without visual/aural cues			N_0	R_3	I_4	C_5	

Copyright © Holly Tuesday Baxter, Julie Allis Berghofer, Lesa MacEwan, Judy Nelson, Kasi Peters, and Penny Roberts 2007

IMTAP - Cognitive

Client Name: _____   **Assessment Date(s):** _____

Rating Scale:
N = Never = 0%   R = Rarely = Under 50%   I = Inconsistent = 50–79%   C = Consistent = 80–100%

E. Long-term Recall (continued)						
viii. Plays intermediate accompaniment without visual/aural cues				N_0	R_4	I_5	C_6
ix. Plays advanced accompaniment without visual/aural cues				N_0	R_4	I_5	C_6
Column Totals:						
Add Column Totals to calculate *Raw Score*:						

Activities/Notes

F. Academics						n/a ☐
i. Matches three colors	N_0	R_2	I_3	C_4		
ii. Matches three symbols	N_0	R_2	I_3	C_4		
iii. Identifies three colors		N_0	R_3	I_4	C_5	
iv. Cued by written symbol to complete or begin task		N_0	R_3	I_4	C_5	
v. Reads simple chord chart		N_0	R_3	I_4	C_5	
vi. Demonstrates understanding of number concepts 1-6		N_0	R_3	I_4	C_5	
vii. Identifies letters A-G		N_0	R_3	I_4	C_5	
viii. Plays simple accompaniment using chord chart *CD*		N_0	R_3	I_4	C_5	
ix. Plays simple melody using written letter cues		N_0	R_3	I_4	C_5	
x. Reads lyrics			N_0	R_4	I_5	C_6
xi. Demonstrates ability to write lyrics			N_0	R_4	I_5	C_6
xii. Reads treble clef notation *CD*			N_0	R_4	I_5	C_6
xiii. Reads bass clef notation			N_0	R_4	I_5	C_6
xiv. Reads bass and treble clef together			N_0	R_4	I_5	C_6
xv. Transcribes musical ideas using symbols or notation *CD*			N_0	R_4	I_5	C_6
Column Totals:						
Add Column Totals to calculate *Raw Score*:						

Activities/Notes

Copyright © Holly Tuesday Baxter, Julie Allis Berghofer, Lesa MacEwan, Judy Nelson, Kasi Peters, and Penny Roberts 2007

IMTAP - Cognitive

Client Name: _____ **Assessment Date(s):** _____

Summary

Sub-Domain	n/a	Raw Score	Possible			Final Score
A. Fundamentals	■		÷	10	=	%
B. Decision Making			÷	18	=	%
C. Direction Following			÷	11	=	%
D. Short-term Recall/Sequencing			÷	11	=	%
E. Long-term Recall			÷	42	=	%
F. Academics			÷	79	=	%
Domain Total (Cognitive)			÷		=	%

CD = Cross Domain Skills

Copyright © Holly Tuesday Baxter, Julie Allis Berghofer, Lesa MacEwan, Judy Nelson, Kasi Peters, and Penny Roberts 2007

IMTAP - Emotional

Client Name: _____   **Assessment Date(s):** _____

Rating Scale:
N = Never = 0%   R = Rarely = Under 50%   I = Inconsistent = 50–79%   C = Consistent = 80–100%

A. Fundamentals							
i.	Demonstrates range of affect		N_0	R_2	I_3	C_4	
ii.	Demonstrates appropriate affect		N_0	R_2	I_3	C_4	
	Column Totals:						
	Add Column Totals to calculate Raw Score:						

Activities/Notes

B. Differentiation/Expression								n/a ☐
i.	Expresses emotions appropriate to circumstances		N_0	R_2	I_3	C_4		
ii.	Expresses emotions using instruments			N_0	R_3	I_4	C_5	
iii.	Expresses emotions verbally			N_0	R_3	I_4	C_5	
iv.	Demonstrates emotional sensitivity to musical components				N_0	R_4	I_5	C_6
	Column Totals:							
	Add Column Totals to calculate Raw Score:							

Activities/Notes

C. Regulation								n/a ☐
i.	Tolerates MT situation without distress		N_0	R_1	I_2	C_3		
ii.	Calms with support *musical/verbal/physical*		N_0	R_1	I_2	C_3		
iii.	Tolerates transitions		N_0	R_1	I_2	C_3		
iv.	Self regulates within one activity			N_0	R_2	I_3	C_4	

Copyright © Holly Tuesday Baxter, Julie Allis Berghofer, Lesa MacEwan, Judy Nelson, Kasi Peters, and Penny Roberts 2007

IMTAP - Emotional

Client Name: _____   **Assessment Date(s):** _____

Rating Scale:
N = Never = 0%   R = Rarely = Under 50%   I = Inconsistent = 50–79%   C = Consistent = 80–100%

C. Regulation (continued)								
v.	Emotional states fluctuate appropriately				N_0	R_2	I_3	C_4
vi.	Remains regulated when limits are set				N_0	R_2	I_3	C_4
	Column Totals:							
	Add Column Totals to calculate **Raw Score:**							
	Activities/Notes							

D. Self-awareness								n/a ☐
i.	Demonstrates recognition of emotional states				N_0	R_4	I_5	C_6
ii.	Demonstrates ability to explore emotional states				N_0	R_4	I_5	C_6
iii.	Demonstrates ability to discuss emotional states				N_0	R_4	I_5	C_6
iv.	Initiates emotional content appropriately				N_0	R_4	I_5	C_6
v.	Demonstrates desire to better oneself or life circumstance				N_0	R_4	I_5	C_6
	Column Totals:							
	Add Column Totals to calculate **Raw Score:**							
	Activities/Notes							

Summary

Sub-Domain	n/a	Raw Score		Possible		Final Score
A. Fundamentals			÷	8	=	%
B. Differentiation/Expression			÷	20	=	%
C. Regulation			÷	21	=	%
D. Self-awareness			÷	30	=	%
Domain Total (Emotional)			÷		=	%

Copyright © Holly Tuesday Baxter, Julie Allis Berghofer, Lesa MacEwan, Judy Nelson, Kasi Peters, and Penny Roberts 2007

IMTAP - Social

Client Name: _____ **Assessment Date(s):** _____

Rating Scale:
N = Never = 0%   R = Rarely = Under 50%   I = Inconsistent = 50–79%   C = Consistent = 80–100%

A. Fundamentals							
i.	Responds to own name	N_0	R_1	I_2	C_3		
ii.	Demonstrates awareness of therapist	N_0	R_1	I_2	C_3		
iii.	Demonstrates interest in presented activities	N_0	R_1	I_2	C_3		
iv.	Demonstrates joint attention	N_0	R_1	I_2	C_3		
v.	Interacts appropriately with therapist	N_0	R_1	I_2	C_3		
vi.	Uses socially appropriate greeting	N_0	R_1	I_2	C_3		
vii.	Uses socially appropriate goodbye	N_0	R_1	I_2	C_3		
viii.	Uses socially appropriate eye contact	N_0	R_1	I_2	C_3		
ix.	Socially references others	N_0	R_1	I_2	C_3		
x.	Demonstrates understanding of rules and structures *CD*		N_0	R_2	I_3	C_4	
xi.	Demonstrates awareness of appropriate physical space		N_0	R_2	I_3	C_4	
xii.	Demonstrates confidence in MT situation		N_0	R_2	I_3	C_4	
	Column Totals:						
	Add Column Totals to calculate **Raw Score**:						
	Activities/Notes						

B. Participation						n/a ☐
i.	Enters room with minimal prompting	N_0	R_1	I_2	C_3	
ii.	Remains in room for duration of session	N_0	R_1	I_2	C_3	
iii.	Attempts new tasks when given opportunity	N_0	R_1	I_2	C_3	
iv.	Initiates new activity when given opportunity	N_0	R_1	I_2	C_3	
v.	Tolerates transitions	N_0	R_1	I_2	C_3	

Copyright © Holly Tuesday Baxter, Julie Allis Berghofer, Lesa MacEwan, Judy Nelson, Kasi Peters, and Penny Roberts 2007

IMTAP - Social

Client Name: _____   **Assessment Date(s):** _____

Rating Scale:
N = Never = 0%   R = Rarely = Under 50%   I = Inconsistent = 50–79%   C = Consistent = 80–100%

B. Participation (continued) n/a ☐

vi.	Participates in structured activities		N_0	R_2	I_3	C_4	
vii.	Is flexible in developing activities		N_0	R_2	I_3	C_4	
viii.	Extends activities appropriately			N_0	R_3	I_4	C_5
ix.	Works towards identified goals in session				N_0	R_4	I_5	C_6

Column Totals:
Add Column Totals to calculate **Raw Score**:

Activities/Notes

C. Turn-taking n/a ☐

i.	Anticipates own turn	N_0	R_1	I_2	C_3		
ii.	Waits for turn		N_0	R_2	I_3	C_4	
iii.	Sustains turn-taking with prompts		N_0	R_2	I_3	C_4	
iv.	Requests turn when appropriate		N_0	R_2	I_3	C_4	
v.	Sustains turn-taking without prompts			N_0	R_3	I_4	C_5

Column Totals:
Add Column Totals to calculate **Raw Score**:

Activities/Notes

D. Attention n/a ☐

i.	Sustains activity length attention span *CD*	N_0	R_1	I_2	C_3		
ii.	Demonstrates sustained attention to therapist	N_0	R_1	I_2	C_3		
iii.	Returns to activity after distraction with prompts	N_0	R_1	I_2	C_3		
iv.	Returns to activity after distraction w/out prompts		N_0	R_2	I_3	C_4	

Column Totals:
Add Column Totals to calculate **Raw Score**:

Activities/Notes

Copyright © Holly Tuesday Baxter, Julie Allis Berghofer, Lesa MacEwan, Judy Nelson, Kasi Peters, and Penny Roberts 2007

IMTAP - Social

Client Name: _____   **Assessment Date(s):** _____

Rating Scale:
N = Never = 0%   R = Rarely = Under 50%   I = Inconsistent = 50–79%   C = Consistent = 80–100%

E. Direction Following   n/a ☐

i. Follows one-step verbal direction CD		N_0	R_1	I_2	C_3	
ii. Follows two-step verbal direction CD		N_0	R_2	I_3	C_4	
iii. Follows simple musical cues CD		N_0	R_2	I_3	C_4	
Column Totals:						

Add Column Totals to calculate **Raw Score:** _____

Activities/Notes

F. Relationship Skills   n/a ☐

i. Tolerates direct interaction	N_0	R_1	I_2	C_3		
ii. Tolerates redirection	N_0	R_1	I_2	C_3		
iii. Tolerates musical contact	N_0	R_1	I_2	C_3		
iv. Plays in parallel with therapist		N_0	R_2	I_3	C_4	
v. Plays in imitation of therapist		N_0	R_2	I_3	C_4	
vi. Sustains musical interaction		N_0	R_2	I_3	C_4	
vii. Sustains two-way communication		N_0	R_2	I_3	C_4	
viii. Works cooperatively with therapist		N_0	R_2	I_3	C_4	
ix. Demonstrates flexibility in interactive musical play			N_0	R_3	I_4	C_5
x. Demonstrates flexibility within familiar interactive structure			N_0	R_3	I_4	C_5
xi. Can assume leadership role in activity			N_0	R_3	I_4	C_5
xii. Moves between independent and interdependent skills			N_0	R_3	I_4	C_5
xiii. Able to explore external social relationships				N_0	R_4	I_5	C_6
Column Totals:						

Add Column Totals to calculate **Raw Score:** _____

Activities/Notes

Copyright © Holly Tuesday Baxter, Julie Allis Berghofer, Lesa MacEwan, Judy Nelson, Kasi Peters, and Penny Roberts 2007

IMTAP - Social

Client Name: _____ **Assessment Date(s):** _____

Summary

Sub-Domain	n/a	Raw Score		Possible		Final Score
A. Fundamentals			÷	39	=	%
B. Participation			÷	34	=	%
C. Turn-taking			÷	20	=	%
D. Attention			÷	13	=	%
E. Direction Following			÷	11	=	%
F. Relationship Skills			÷	55	=	%
Domain Total (Social)			÷		=	%

CD = Cross Domain Skills

Copyright © Holly Tuesday Baxter, Julie Allis Berghofer, Lesa MacEwan, Judy Nelson, Kasi Peters, and Penny Roberts 2007

IMTAP - Musicality

Client Name: _____   **Assessment Date(s):** _____

Rating Scale:
N = Never = 0%   R = Rarely = Under 50%   I = Inconsistent = 50–79%   C = Consistent = 80–100%

A. Fundamentals						
i. Is alerted by music	N_0	R_1	I_2	C_3		
ii. Expresses enjoyment of music	N_0	R_1	I_2	C_3		
iii. Indicates desire to play/touch instruments	N_0	R_1	I_2	C_3		
iv. Plays instrument when presented	N_0	R_1	I_2	C_3		
v. Explores instruments	N_0	R_1	I_2	C_3		
vi. Vocalizes in response to music	N_0	R_1	I_2	C_3		
vii. Moves rhythmically in response to music	N_0	R_1	I_2	C_3		
viii. Plays instruments spontaneously	N_0	R_1	I_2	C_3		
ix. Sings spontaneously		N_0	R_2	I_3	C_4	
x. Responds to simple musical cue		N_0	R_2	I_3	C_4	
xi. Engages in interactive musical play		N_0	R_2	I_3	C_4	
xii. Regulates with musical support		N_0	R_2	I_3	C_4	
Column Totals:						
Add Column Totals to calculate Raw Score:						

Activities/Notes

B. Tempo							n/a ☐
i. Tolerates changing tempo	N_0	R_1	I_2	C_3			
ii. Demonstrates awareness of gross tempo changes CD	N_0	R_1	I_2	C_3			
iii. Unconscious body movements in tempo CD	N_0	R_1	I_2	C_3			
iv. Conscious body movement in tempo CD	N_0	R_1	I_2	C_3			
v. Plays in own tempo 1–4 measures		N_0	R_2	I_3	C_4		
vi. Plays in tempo of therapist 1–4 measures CD		N_0	R_2	I_3	C_4		
vii. Initiates tempo changes		N_0	R_2	I_3	C_4		
viii. Adapts playing to match tempo changes CD		N_0	R_2	I_3	C_4		
ix. Adapts playing to follow accelerando		N_0	R_2	I_3	C_4		
x. Sustains playing in own tempo interactively		N_0	R_2	I_3	C_4		
xi. Sustains playing in tempo of therapist interactively			N_0	R_3	I_4	C_5	

Copyright © Holly Tuesday Baxter, Julie Allis Berghofer, Lesa MacEwan, Judy Nelson, Kasi Peters, and Penny Roberts 2007

IMTAP - Musicality

Client Name: _____   **Assessment Date(s):** _____

Rating Scale:
N = Never = 0%   R = Rarely = Under 50%   I = Inconsistent = 50–79%   C = Consistent = 80–100%

B. Tempo (continued)

xii. Plays multiples of basic beat				N_0	R_4	I_5	C_6
xiii. Adapts playing to follow ritardando				N_0	R_4	I_5	C_6
Column Totals:						
Add Column Totals to calculate **Raw Score:**						

Activities/Notes

C. Rhythm   n/a ☐

i. Imitates simple rhythmic pattern CD	N_0	R_2	I_3	C_4		
ii. Imitates intermediate rhythmic pattern CD	N_0	R_2	I_3	C_4		
iii. Beats rhythmic pattern of melody or words		N_0	R_3	I_4	C_5	
iv. Sustains imitation of varying rhythmic patterns		N_0	R_3	I_4	C_5	
v. Changes rhythmic pattern in response to music			N_0	R_4	I_5	C_6
vi. Coordinates two differing rhythmic patterns			N_0	R_4	I_5	C_6
vii. Initiates differing rhythmic patterns during turn taking			N_0	R_4	I_5	C_6
viii. Initiates rhythmic structures involving multiple patterns			N_0	R_4	I_5	C_6
ix. Develops rhythmic structures involving multiple patterns			N_0	R_4	I_5	C_6
x. Sustains self-initiated rhythmic patterns			N_0	R_4	I_5	C_6
xi. Adapts playing to match meter changes CD			N_0	R_4	I_5	C_6
Column Totals:						
Add Column Totals to calculate **Raw Score:**						

Activities/Notes

Copyright © Holly Tuesday Baxter, Julie Allis Berghofer, Lesa MacEwan, Judy Nelson, Kasi Peters, and Penny Roberts 2007

IMTAP - Musicality

Client Name: _____   Assessment Date(s): _____

Rating Scale:
N = Never = 0%   R = Rarely = Under 50%   I = Inconsistent = 50–79%   C = Consistent = 80–100%

D. Dynamics n/a ☐

i.	Demonstrates awareness of gross dynamic changes CD	N_0	R_1	I_2	C_3		
ii.	Tolerates changing dynamic	N_0	R_1	I_2	C_3		
iii.	Demonstrates variety of dynamics in playing		N_0	R_2	I_3	C_4	
iv.	Initiates dynamic changes		N_0	R_2	I_3	C_4	
v.	Follows cue to change dynamic		N_0	R_2	I_3	C_4	
vi.	Adapts playing to crescendo		N_0	R_2	I_3	C_4	
vii.	Adapts playing to diminuendo			N_0	R_3	I_4	C_5
viii.	Demonstrates control of crescendo				N_0	R_4	I_5	C_6
ix.	Demonstrates control of diminuendo				N_0	R_4	I_5	C_6
x.	Demonstrates expressive use of diminuendo/crescendo				N_0	R_4	I_5	C_6

Column Totals:
Add Column Totals to calculate Raw Score:

Activities/Notes

E. Vocal n/a ☐

i.	Unconscious vocalizations in tonality CD	N_0	R_1	I_2	C_3		
ii.	Vocalizes in response to particular musical style/idiom CD	N_0	R_1	I_2	C_3		
iii.	Communicative vocalizations in tonality of music		N_0	R_2	I_3	C_4	
iv.	Vocalizes to complete known song phrase		N_0	R_2	I_3	C_4	
v.	Sings in key or tonality		N_0	R_2	I_3	C_4	
vi.	Sings pitched melody accurately CD		N_0	R_2	I_3	C_4	
vii.	Sings using sensitivity to musical components			N_0	R_3	I_4	C_5
viii.	Sings in round				N_0	R_4	I_5	C_6

Copyright © Holly Tuesday Baxter, Julie Allis Berghofer, Lesa MacEwan, Judy Nelson, Kasi Peters, and Penny Roberts 2007

IMTAP - Musicality

Client Name: _____   **Assessment Date(s):** _____

Rating Scale:
N = Never = 0%   R = Rarely = Under 50%   I = Inconsistent = 50–79%   C = Consistent = 80–100%

E. Vocal (continued)

ix.	Sings harmony line				N_0	R_4	I_5	C_6
x.	Sings expressing lyric content and meaning				N_0	R_4	I_5	C_6
xi.	Creates self expressive lyrical improvisation				N_0	R_4	I_5	C_6
xii.	Creates and sings own song structure				N_0	R_4	I_5	C_6

Column Totals:

Add Column Totals to calculate Raw Score:

Activities/Notes

F. Perfect and Relative Pitch   n/a ☐

i.	Seeks and matches single tones				N_0	R_3	I_4	C_5	
ii.	Plays melodically in tonality of music				N_0	R_4	I_5	C_6
iii.	Identifies letter name of tone or key per aural cue				N_0	R_4	I_5	C_6
iv.	Initiates song in original key				N_0	R_4	I_5	C_6
v.	Plays known melody by ear				N_0	R_4	I_5	C_6
vi.	Changes key to match changing tonality				N_0	R_4	I_5	C_6
vii.	Transposes music by ear				N_0	R_4	I_5	C_6

Column Totals:

Add Column Totals to calculate Raw Score:

Activities/Notes

G. Creativity and Development of Musical Ideas   n/a ☐

i.	Creates melody independently	N_0	R_2	I_3	C_4	
ii.	Improvises melody to given rhythmic pattern	N_0	R_2	I_3	C_4	
iii.	Assigns differentiated instruments to given ideas or images		N_0	R_3	I_4	C_5
iv.	Assigns differentiated musical motifs to given ideas or images.		N_0	R_3	I_4	C_5

Copyright © Holly Tuesday Baxter, Julie Allis Berghofer, Lesa MacEwan, Judy Nelson, Kasi Peters, and Penny Roberts 2007

IMTAP - Musicality

Client Name: _____   **Assessment Date(s):** _____

Rating Scale:
N = Never = 0%   R = Rarely = Under 50%   I = Inconsistent = 50–79%   C = Consistent = 80–100%

G. *Creativity and Development of Musical Ideas (continued)*							
v. Creates music to poem or story			N_0	R_3	I_4	C_5	
vi. Improvises words to given rhythmic pattern			N_0	R_3	I_4	C_5	
vii. Improvises rhythmic structure			N_0	R_3	I_4	C_5	
viii. Initiates phrase length musical idea in call and response			N_0	R_3	I_4	C_5	
ix. Creates melodic phrase with harmonic support			N_0	R_3	I_4	C_5	
x. Improvises harmony				N_0	R_4	I_5	C_6
xi. Extends known structure through improvisation				N_0	R_4	I_5	C_6
xii. Creates complete song structure				N_0	R_4	I_5	C_6
xiii. Transcribes musical ideas using symbols or notation *CD*				N_0	R_4	I_5	C_6
xiv. Improvises expressively using musical components				N_0	R_4	I_5	C_6
xv. Improvises in recognizable musical style				N_0	R_4	I_5	C_6
xvi. Improvises in recognizable musical mode				N_0	R_4	I_5	C_6
xvii. Creates self expressive improvisation				N_0	R_4	I_5	C_6

Column Totals: ____

Add Column Totals to calculate Raw Score: ____

Activities/Notes

H. **Music Reading**							n/a ☐
i. Plays simple accompaniment using chord chart *CD*			N_0	R_3	I_4	C_5	
ii. Reads and plays simple rhythmic notation			N_0	R_3	I_4	C_5	
iii. Plays melody of song from written cues				N_0	R_4	I_5	C_6
iv. Reads treble clef notation *CD*				N_0	R_4	I_5	C_6
v. Reads and plays music in treble clef notation				N_0	R_4	I_5	C_6
vi. Reads bass clef notation				N_0	R_4	I_5	C_6
vii. Reads and plays music in bass clef notation				N_0	R_4	I_5	C_6

Rating Scale:

Copyright © Holly Tuesday Baxter, Julie Allis Berghofer, Lesa MacEwan, Judy Nelson, Kasi Peters, and Penny Roberts 2007

IMTAP - Musicality

Client Name: _____   **Assessment Date(s):** _____

N = Never = 0%   R = Rarely = Under 50%   I = Inconsistent = 50–79%   C = Consistent = 80–100%

H. Music Reading (continued)

viii. Simultaneously reads and plays melody and chords				N_0	R_4	I_5	C_6
ix. Reads and plays bass and treble clef together				N_0	R_4	I_5	C_6
Column Totals:							

Add Column Totals to calculate **Raw Score:** _____

Activities/Notes

I. Accompaniment   n/a ☐

i. Accompanies therapist singing/playing		N_0	R_2	I_3	C_4	
ii. Vocalizes and plays simultaneously with pulse		N_0	R_3	I_4	C_5	
iii. Accompanies self with harmonic instrument		N_0	R_4	I_5	C_6	
Column Totals:						

Add Column Totals to calculate **Raw Score:** _____

Activities/Notes

Copyright © Holly Tuesday Baxter, Julie Allis Berghofer, Lesa MacEwan, Judy Nelson, Kasi Peters, and Penny Roberts 2007

IMTAP - Musicality

Client Name: _____   **Assessment Date(s):** _____

Summary

Sub-Domain	n/a	Raw Score	Possible			Final Score
A. Fundamentals	▓		÷	40	=	%
B. Tempo			÷	53	=	%
C. Rhythm			÷	60	=	%
D. Dynamics			÷	45	=	%
E. Vocal			÷	57	=	%
F. Perfect and Relative Pitch			÷	41	=	%
G. Creativity and Development of Musical Ideas/Vocal and Instrumental			÷	91	=	%
H. Music Reading			÷	52	=	%
I. Accompaniment			÷	15	=	%
Domain Total (Musicality)			÷		=	%

CD = Cross Domain Skills

Copyright © Holly Tuesday Baxter, Julie Allis Berghofer, Lesa MacEwan, Judy Nelson, Kasi Peters, and Penny Roberts 2007

Individualized Music Therapy Assessment Profile (IMTAP)
Summary

Client: _____ D.O.B./Age: _____

Music Therapist: _____

Date(s) of Assessment: _____ Date to be Reviewed: _____

STRENGTHS:

NEEDS:

_____
Music Therapist Signature   Date

Copyright © Holly Tuesday Baxter, Julie Allis Berghofer, Lesa MacEwan, Judy Nelson, Kasi Peters, and Penny Roberts 2007

Individualized Music Therapy Assessment Profile (IMTAP)
Goals and Objectives

Client: _____ D.O.B./Age: _____

Music Therapist: _____

Date: _____ Date to be Reviewed: _____

GOAL # ___

☐ Gross Motor ☐ Fine Motor ☐ Oral Motor ☐ Sensory ☐ Receptive Communication/Auditory Perception
☐ Expressive Communication ☐ Cognitive ☐ Emotional ☐ Social

Goal: _____

_____ *Date reached*: _____

Objective A: _____

_____ *Date reached*: _____

Objective B: _____

_____ *Date reached*: _____

GOAL # ___

☐ Gross Motor ☐ Fine Motor ☐ Oral Motor ☐ Sensory ☐ Receptive Communication/Auditory Perception
☐ Expressive Communication ☐ Cognitive ☐ Emotional ☐ Social

Goal: _____

_____ *Date reached*: _____

Objective A: _____

_____ *Date reached*: _____

Objective B: _____

_____ *Date reached*: _____

_____   _____
Music Therapist Signature   Date

Copyright © Holly Tuesday Baxter, Julie Allis Berghofer, Lesa MacEwan, Judy Nelson, Kasi Peters, and Penny Roberts 2007

Individualized Music Therapy Assessment Profile (IMTAP)

Client Name: _____ **Date of Birth:** _____ **Assessment Date(s):** _____

Title: _____ **Type of graph:** ☐ Domain Profile ☐ Sub-domain Profile

Domain/Sub-domain	0%	10%	20%	30%	40%	50%	60%	70%	80%	90%	100%

Copyright © Holly Tuesday Baxter, Julie Allis Berghofer, Lesa MacEwan, Judy Nelson, Kasi Peters, and Penny Roberts 2007

Individualized Music Therapy Assessment Profile (IMTAP)
Quantification Tally Sheet

Client's Name: _____   Session Date: _____

Skill Observed: _____

Observer: _____   Reliability Observer: _____

Record/Observe Interval (in seconds): _____

1 --:--	Obs	+ V M O A	Obs	+ V M O A	Obs	+ V M O A	Obs	+ V M O A	Obs	+ V M O A	Obs	+ V M O A
2 --:--	Obs	+ V M O A	Obs	+ V M O A	Obs	+ V M O A	Obs	+ V M O A	Obs	+ V M O A	Obs	+ V M O A
3 --:--	Obs	+ V M O A	Obs	+ V M O A	Obs	+ V M O A	Obs	+ V M O A	Obs	+ V M O A	Obs	+ V M O A
4 --:--	Obs	+ V M O A	Obs	+ V M O A	Obs	+ V M O A	Obs	+ V M O A	Obs	+ V M O A	Obs	+ V M O A
5 --:--	Obs	+ V M O A	Obs	+ V M O A	Obs	+ V M O A	Obs	+ V M O A	Obs	+ V M O A	Obs	+ V M O A

+ = Desired skill demonstrated   +: _____ / _____ = _____ %

V = Verbal distraction   V: _____ / _____ = _____ %

M = Motor distraction   M: _____ / _____ = _____ %

O = No interaction; daydreaming, etc. O: _____ / _____ = _____ %

A = n/a   A: _____ / _____ = _____ %

This form is modeled after an observation form found in *Teaching/Discipline: A Positive Approach for Educational Development. 4th ed*, by Clifford K. Madsen and Charles H. Madsen Jr, Contemporary Publishing Company, Raleigh, NC. It is used by permission.

Copyright © Holly Tuesday Baxter, Julie Allis Berghofer, Lesa MacEwan, Judy Nelson, Kasi Peters, and Penny Roberts 2007

Appendix B

Music Reading Samples

IMTAP Music Sample Hii
Reads and plays simple rhythmic notation

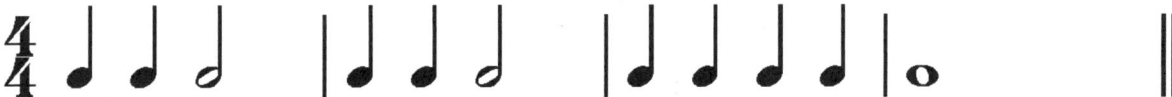

OR

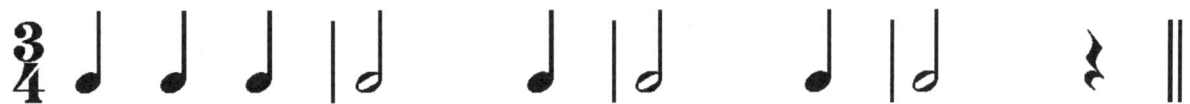

Copyright © Holly Tuesday Baxter, Julie Allis Berghofer, Lesa MacEwan, Judy Nelson, Kasi Peters, and Penny Roberts 2007

IMTAP Music Sample Hiii
Plays melody of song from written cues

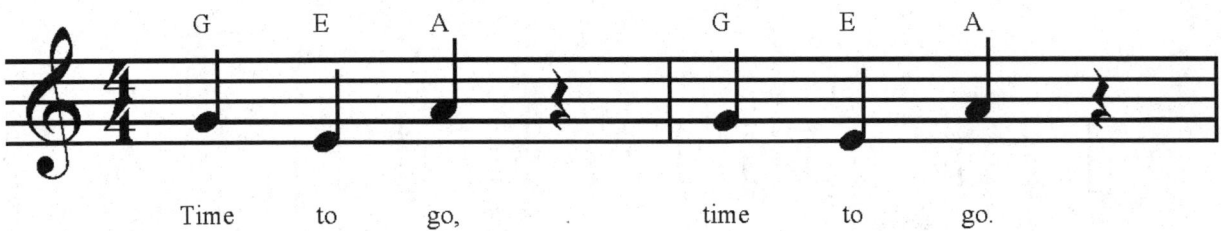

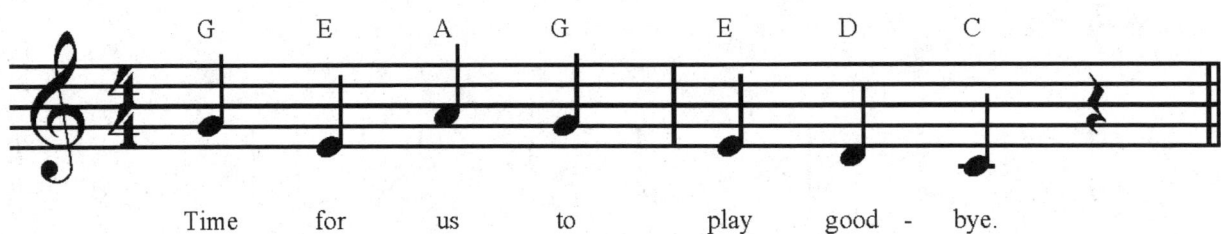

Copyright © Holly Tuesday Baxter, Julie Allis Berghofer, Lesa MacEwan, Judy Nelson, Kasi Peters, and Penny Roberts 2007

IMTAP Music Sample Hv
Reads and plays music in treble clef notation

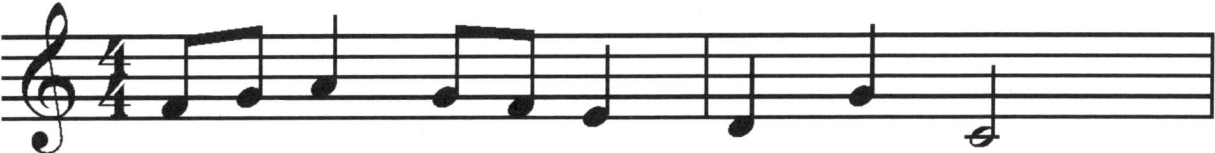

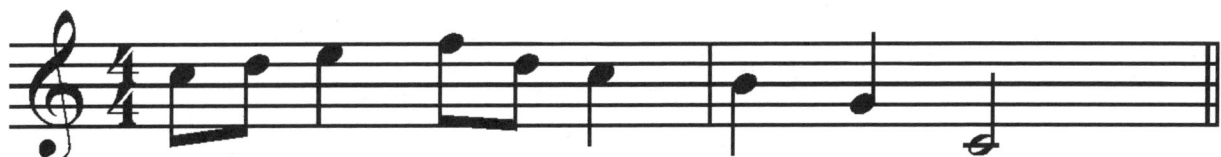

Copyright © Holly Tuesday Baxter, Julie Allis Berghofer, Lesa MacEwan, Judy Nelson, Kasi Peters, and Penny Roberts 2007

IMTAP Music Sample Hvii
Reads and plays music in bass clef notation

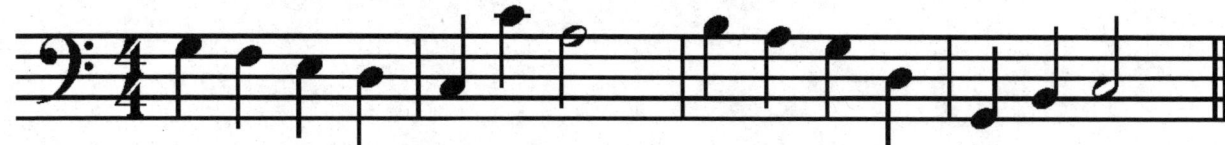

Copyright © Holly Tuesday Baxter, Julie Allis Berghofer, Lesa MacEwan, Judy Nelson, Kasi Peters, and Penny Roberts 2007

IMTAP Music Sample Hix
Reads and plays bass and treble clef together

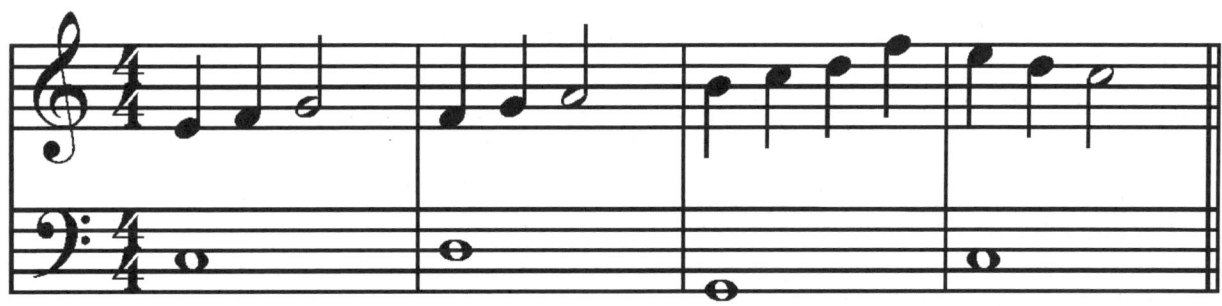

Copyright © Holly Tuesday Baxter, Julie Allis Berghofer, Lesa MacEwan, Judy Nelson, Kasi Peters, and Penny Roberts 2007

References

Alley, J. M. (1979) "Music in the IEP: Therapy/education." *Journal of Music Therapy 16*, 3, 111–127.

American Music Therapy Association (2005) In A. Elkins (ed) *AMTA Member Sourcebook 2005*. Silver Spring, MD: American Music Therapy Association.

Bruscia, K. (1989) *Defining Music Therapy*. Phoenixville, PA: Barcelona Publishers.

Chase, K. M. (2004) "Music Therapy Assessment for Children with Developmental Disabilities: A Survey Study." *Journal of Music Therapy 24*, 1, 28–54.

Cohen, G., Auerbach, J., and Katz, E. (1978) "Music Therapy Assessment of the Developmentally Disabled Client." *Journal of Music Therapy 15*, 2, 88–99.

Davis, W. B., Gfeller, K. E., and Thaut, M. H. (1999) *An Introduction to Music Therapy Theory and Practice*. New York: McGraw-Hill.

Downing, J. E. (1996) *Including Students with Severe and Multiple Disabilities in Typical Classrooms: Practical Strategies for Teachers*. Baltimore: Brookes.

Elliott, J., Ysseldyke, J., Thurlow, M., and Erickson, R. (1998) "What About Assessment and Accountability? Practical Implications for Educators." *Teaching Exceptional Children 31*, 1, 20–27.

Flowers, C., Ahlgrim-Delzell, L., Browder, D., and Spooner, F. (2005) "Teachers' Perceptions of Alternate Assessments." *Research and Practice for Persons with Severe Disabilities 30*, 2, 81–92.

Gantt, L. (2000) "Assessments in the Creative Arts Therapies: Learning from Each Other." *Music Therapy Perspectives 18*, 1, 41–46.

Gaston, E. T. (1968) *Music in Therapy*. New York: Macmillan.

Grant, R. E. (1995) "Music Therapy Assessment for Developmentally Disabled Clients." In T. Wigram, B. Saperston, and R. West (eds) *The Art and Science of Music Therapy: A Handbook* (pp.273–287). Switzerland: Harwood Academic Publishers.

Gregory, D. (2000) "Test instruments used by Journal of Music Therapy authors from 1984–1997." *Journal of Music Therapy 37*, 2, 79–94.

Gunning, T. G. (2000) *Creating Literacy Instruction for All Children*, 3rd ed. Boston, MA: Allyn and Bacon.

Hintz, M. R. (2000) "Geriatric Music Therapy Clinical Assessment: Assessment of Music Skills and Related Behaviors." *Music Therapy Perspectives 18*, 1, 31–40.

Individuals with Disabilities Education Act Amendments of 2004, PL 108–446, 118 Stat. 2647 (2004). Washington, D.C.: US Department of Education. Accessed on 3 October 2007 at http://nichcy.org/reauth/PL108-446.pdf

Isenberg-Grzeda, C. (1988) "Music Therapy Assessment: A Reflection of Professional Identity." *Journal of Music Therapy 25*, 3, 156–169.

James, M. R., Weaver, A. L., Clemens, P. D., and Plaster, G. A. (1985) "Influence of Paired Auditory and Vestibular Stimulation on Levels of Motor Skill Development in a Mentally Retarded Population." *Journal of Music Therapy 21*, 4, 22–34.

REFERENCES

Lipe, A. W. (1995) "The use of music performance tasks in the assessment of cognitive functioning among older adults with dementia." *Journal of Music Therapy 32*, 3, 137–51.

No Child Left Behind Act of 2001, PL 107–110, 115 Stat. 1425 (2002). Washington, D.C.: US Department of Education. Accessed on 3 October 2007 at www.ed.gov/policy/elsec/leg/esea02/107-110.pdf

Nordoff, P. and Robbins, C. (1985) *Therapy in Music for Handicapped Children.* London: Gollancz.

Orelove, F. P. and Sobsey, D. (1996) *Educating Children with Multiple Disabilities: A Transdisciplinary Approach*, 3rd ed. Baltimore: Paul H. Brookes.

Scalenghe, R. and Murphy, K. M. (2000) "Music Therapy Assessment in the Managed Care Environment." *Music Therapy Perspectives 18*, 1, 23–30.

Shuter-Dyson, R. (1982) "Musical Ability." In D. Deutsch (ed) *The Psychology of Music* (pp.391–412). New York: Academic Press.

Standley, J. M. and Hughes, J. E. (1997) "Evaluation of an Early Intervention Music Curriculum for Enhancing Prereading/Writing Skills. *Music Therapy Perspectives 15*, 2, 79–85.

Thompson, A. B., Arnold, J. C., and Murray, S. E. (1990) "Music Therapy Assessment of the Cerebrovascular Patient." *Music Therapy Perspectives 8*, 23–29.

Westling, D. L. and Fox, L. (2004) *Teaching Students with Severe Disabilities*, 3rd ed. Upper Saddle River: Prentice-Hall.

Wigram, T. (2000) "A Method of Music Therapy Assessment for the Diagnosis of Autism and Communication Disorders in Children." *Music Therapy Perspectives 18*, 1, 13–22.

Wilson, B. L. and Smith, D. S. (2000) "Music Therapy Assessment in School Settings: A Preliminary Investigation." *Journal of Music Therapy 37*, 2, 95–117.

Index

academic skills 68–70
accompaniment 91
accountability 17, 18, 20
administration
   instructions 25–36
   time, step-by-step process 14–15
age-appropriate interpretation of
   scores 25–6
age-appropriate language 26
air production 51
Alley, J. M. 19, 20
American Music Therapy Association
   (AMTA) 17
answering questions 64, 66
Arnold, J. C. 19
assessment
   necessity of 17
   process 26–36
attention 76
auditory skills 56–7
   transposition 87
   see also receptive
      communication/auditory
      perception (RC)
Auerbach, J. 18
autoharp/Q Chord 47–8

bass clef notation 70, 91
benefits of IMTAP 13–14
Board Certified Music Therapists 15
Bruscia, K. 19

case studies 93–126
   Neil 93–107
   Timothy 108–26
Chase, K. M. 17, 18, 19
chord charts 48, 69, 70, 90
chords 48, 91
cognitive (COG) skills 23, 65–70
   academic 68–70

decision making 66
direction following 66–7
fundamentals 65
long-term recall 67–8
short-term recall/sequencing 67
Cohen, G. 18
colors 68, 69
communication
   non-vocal 61–2
   relational 63
   see also expressive communication
      (EC); receptive
      communication/auditory
      perception (RC); social (SOC)
      skills; verbalizations;
      vocalizations
computer software 14, 15, 127–34
   installing 127–8
   using 128–34
   see also scoring
coordination 44, 47, 48
   of differing rhythm patterns 83
cover sheet 14, 28
creativity and development of ideas
   87–90
cross-domain skills review 31–3
cues, responding to 45
   musical 57, 58, 66, 67, 77, 80, 87
   written 68, 69, 70, 90

data collection 28–36, 39–41
Davis, W. B. 18
decision making 66
development of IMTAP 21–4
diagnosis-appropriate language 26
differentiation, emotional skills 71
direction following 62, 66–7, 77
disabilities, children with
   accountability for 17

qualities of music therapy
   assessment 19–20
distractions
   recording 39–40
   returning to task following 54, 55,
      56–7, 76
domain profile graph 34–5
domain scoring forms 14, 15
domains and sub-domains of IMTAP
   22–4
   see also specific domains
Downing, J. E. 17
dulcimer/guitar skills 48
dynamics 84–5
   changes 45, 58

Elliot, J. 17
emotional (EMO) skills 23, 71–3
   differentiation/expression 71
   fundamentals 71
   regulation 71–2
   self-awareness 72–3
enjoyment of music 79
estimated scores 29
expression, emotional 71
expressive communication (EC) 23,
   61–5
   fundamentals 61
   non-vocal communication 61–2
   relational communication 63
   see also verbalizations; vocalizations

features of IMTAP 13–14
fine motor (FM) skills 22, 45–50
   autoharp/Q Chord 47–8
   fundamentals 45–6
   guitar/dulcimer 48
   piano 48–50
   pitched percussive/mallet 50
   strumming 47

INDEX

and tone production, oral motor skills 51
Flowers, C. 17
Fox, L. 17

Gantt, L. 18
Gaston, E. T. 20
gestures and vocalizations, combining 58
Gfeller, K. E. 18
goals and objectives
 computer software 132–3
 form 14, 34
Grant, R. E. 18, 19, 20
graphing 34–6
Gregory, D. 18
gross motor (GM) skills 22, 43–5
 fundamentals 43–4
 perceptual/visual/psycho motor 44–5
 and tone production, oral motor skills 51
guitar/dulcimer skills 48
Gunning, T. G. 17

hands
 left/right dominance 43, 45, 49, 50
 movements 45–50
 tactile skills 52–3
harmony 89
head
 orientation in space 54
 turning to sound source 57
Hintz, M. R. 18
history of IMTAP 21
Hughes, J. E. 19

ideas, creativity and development of 87–90
imitation
 movements 44
 musical motifs 57, 60, 76
 rhythmic pattern 82
 vocalizations 59–60, 62
improvisation 87, 88
Individualized Education Programs (IEPs) 19
Individualized Music Therapy Assessment Profile (IMTAP) 11–12, 13–15, 21–4

Individuals with Disabilities Education Act Amendments 2004 (IDEA) 17
initial contact 26
initiation 73, 75, 81, 83, 84, 87, 88
 of verbal discussion 60, 73
intake
 computer software 130–1
 form 14, 26–7
interdisciplinary teams 18, 20, 21
Isenberg-Grzeda, C. 18, 20
item development of IMTAP 21

James, M. R. 19

Katz, E. 18

left/right dominance 43, 45, 49, 50
letters, identification of 69, 87
Lipe, A. W. 18
long-term recall 67–8
lyrics 70, 86, 88, 89
 expressing content and meaning 86

mallet skills 50
melody 63, 64, 70, 85, 87
 and harmony 89
 music reading 90, 91
meter changes 45, 63, 84
motivation 19
mouthpieces 51, 53
movement 43, 44
 imitation 44
 in response to music 79, 80
 sequences 45, 49, 50
multi-sensory medium of music 19
Murphy, K. M. 18, 19
Murray, S. E. 19
music reading 90–1
Music Therapy Wellness Clinic 11
musical changes 58–9
 dynamics 45, 58
 meter 45, 58, 84
 pitch 62
 tempo 45, 62, 80, 81
musical cues, responding to 57, 58, 66, 67, 77, 80, 87
musicality (MUS) 24, 79–91
 accompaniment 91
 creativity and development of ideas 87–90
 dynamics 84–5

fundamentals 79–80
music reading 90–1
perfect and relative pitch 86–7
rhythm 82–4
tempo 80–1
vocal 85–6

need for assessment 17, 18–19
Neil (case study) 93–107
No Child Left Behind Act 2001 (NCLB) 17
non-assessed sub-domains and skills 29
non-verbal aspect of music 19–20
non-vocal communication 61–2
Nordoff, P. 20
notation/symbols 69, 70, 89, 90–1
number concepts 69

observation and recording *see* recording
oral motor (OM) skills 22, 50–1
 air production 51
 fundamentals 50
Orelove, F. P. 17

palmar grasp 46
parent/guardian issues 26, 27
participation, social (SOC) skills 74–5
percussive instruments 50
perfect and relative pitch 86–7
piano skills 48–50
pincer grasp 46
pitch
 changes 58
 perfect and relative 86–7
 range 62
pitched instruments
 percussive/mallet skills 50
 vocalizing response to 59
proprioceptive skills 53–4
purpose of IMTAP 13

Q Chord/autoharp 47–8
qualities of assessment 19–20
quantification module 14, 37–41
 preparation 37–9
questions, responding to 64, 66

rapport, establishing 26
rationale, music therapy as assessment protocol 17–20

recall 67–8
receptive communication/auditory
    perception (RC) 23, 57–60
  direction following 57–8
  fundamentals 57
  rhythm 60
  singing/vocalizing 59–60
  see also musical changes
recording 25, 26
  computer software 129, 131–3
  and observing 38, 39–40
Registered Music Therapists 15
regulation of emotions 71–2
relational communication 63
relationship skills 77–8
reports 134
reviewing cross-domain skills 31–3
rhythm 60, 82–4
  improvisation 87, 88
  movement in response to music 79
  production, oral motor skills 51
Robbins, C. 20

Scalenghe, R. 18, 19
scoring 24, 28–31, 38–9
  age-appropriate 25–6
  domain scoring forms 14, 15
  tallying 29, 39, 40, 41
self-awareness 72–3
sensory (SEN) skills 22, 52–7
  auditory 56–7
  fundamentals 52
  proprioceptive 53–4
  tactile 52–3
  vestibular 54
  visual 55
sequences, movement 45, 49, 50
sequencing 67
session outline form 14, 28
session planning 15, 25, 26
short-term recall 67
Shuter-Dyson, R. 19
singing/songs *see* lyrics; vocalizations
skills
  definitions 43–91
  selection 37–8
social (SOC) skills 23, 73–8
  attention 76
  direction following 77
  fundamentals 73–4
  participation 74–5
  relationship 77–8
  turn-taking 75–6

Smith, D. S. 18
spontaneous vocalizations 62–3
Sobsey, D. 17
Standley, J. M. 19
strumming skills 47
sub-domain profile graph 35–6
sub-domains of IMTAP 22–4
  and skills, non-assessed 29
summary sheet 14, 34
symbols/notation 69, 70, 89, 90–1

tactile skills 52–3
tempo 44, 60, 80–1
  changes 45, 58, 80
Thaut, M. H. 18
Thompson, A. B. 19
time cueing system 38
Timothy (case study) 108–26
tonality 58–9, 85, 86, 87
tone production, oral motor skills 51
treble clef notation 70, 90, 91
turn-taking 75–6

user qualifications 15

verbal directions, following 57–8,
  66, 77
verbalizations 63
  of emotional states 71, 72–3
  initiation 60, 73
vestibular skills 54
visual skills 44–5, 55
  orientation to sound source 57
vocalizations 62
  accompaniment 91
  answering questions 64, 66
  and gestures, combining 62
  idiosyncrasies 64–5
  musicality (MUS) 85–6
  receptive communication/auditory
    perception (RC) 57–60
  responses 57–8, 79, 80
  spontaneous 62–3

Westling, D. L. 17
Wigram, T. 19
Wilson, B. L. 18
written cues, responding to 68, 69,
  70, 90